NEW DISCOVERIES IN MEDICINE

BAMPTON LECTURES IN AMERICA · *Number 2*

DELIVERED AT COLUMBIA UNIVERSITY

1 9 4 9

NEW DISCOVERIES IN MEDICINE

Their Effect on the Public Health

by PAUL R. HAWLEY

Essay Index Reprint Series

Originally Published by
COLUMBIA UNIVERSITY PRESS
NEW YORK

 BOOKS FOR LIBRARIES PRESS
FREEPORT, NEW YORK

Library of Congress Cataloging in Publication Data

Hawley, Paul R   1891-1965.
    New discoveries in medicine.

    (Essay index reprint series)
    1. Medicine--Addresses, essays, lectures. I. Title.
 ₍R708.H4   1972₎   610   76-37922
 ISBN 0-8369-2594-7

PRINTED IN THE UNITED STATES OF AMERICA
BY
NEW WORLD BOOK MANUFACTURING CO., INC.
HALLANDALE, FLORIDA 33009

PREFACE

W HEN THIS UNIVERSITY honored me with the invitation to give the Bampton Lectures in America, the Acting President, while graciously permitting me a free choice of topics, suggested that a series of talks upon the general theme of new discoveries in the field of medicine and their effect upon the public health might be both timely and of general interest.

I agreed readily with this suggestion, having in mind no other theme which interested me more and knowing that there is no scarcity of material in this field.

It was with a growing sense of anxiety, however, that I explored the field. Instead of making my labors less arduous, the very abundance of material made them greater. I know of no more worrisome task than that of selecting a few choice items from a large assortment of attractive offerings, whether this be at the dinner table, a gift shop, or the race track.

Then there was the question of whether a generous helping of a few delicacies would be more or less satisfying than numerous small portions of many. After some deliberation, the former course was selected in the hope that it would leave with the audiences a fair degree of understanding of these phenomena rather than fleeting impressions of a crazy quilt of many patterns.

Another decision to be made was the limit to be placed upon "new" as it is applied to discoveries in the field of medicine. "New" is a relative term, the limit of which is related to the field in which it is applied. A new hairdo is one thing; a new upheaval of the earth's crust is another. Medicine is a very ancient art, and a discovery within a current century cannot be said to be old. I have, however, dipped into ancient medical history only when it seemed to me that such a background added to the interest; and I have included work done a quarter-century ago when I considered the origins of present-day advances essential to a clear understanding.

Some may wonder why I have passed over the discoveries in the antibiotics and other drugs which have revolutionized the treatment of infections of all kinds. It is probable that the influence they are exerting upon the public health is more profound than that of any other innovation of the past century. It seemed to me, however, that there is little to be said about these discoveries that would be of interest to listeners not associated with biology, biochemistry, or vital statistics. There are certain chemicals which are tolerated by the human body in doses that are lethal to some pathogenic microorganisms. Some species of free-living molds are already known, and others are being discovered, which, in their metabolism produce substances that kill bacteria or viruses or both. Having said this much, one cannot go farther without becoming involved in complex chemical formulae and in immunological phenomena which are not yet fully understood.

The circulatory system offers a much more productive field for interesting the nonmedical person. Much of its operation is governed by mechanical principles encountered in everyday life. Many of its biochemical reactions can be illustrated by the application of common experience.

The blood is almost a world unto itself. In it, strange things happen constantly—some that are beneficial, and some that are deleterious to health. It is not necessary to understand the chemistry of these phenomena to comprehend the mechanics—if such a term be permissible. Some of the most important advances of the day are being made in the field of hematology and in the physiology and pathology of the circulatory system, with the promise of more to come in the future; and so the circulatory system seemed to lend itself to discussions of this nature.

No series of talks upon this general theme would be complete without some mention of the great advances in the understanding and the treatment of mental illnesses—advances that are very great when compared with the ineffectual gropings of thousands of years. Much of the advance in the cure of physical ills has come through animal experimentation. In such research, an actual living body can be subjected to innumerable controlled conditions. Except for limited use in psychological experimentation, animals cannot contribute much to the study of mental processes. The mind cannot be laid open for visual observation and study as can be the digestive tract. The obstacles to psychiatric research are formidable, and the achievements therein are correspondingly remarkable.

Finally, one of the most important issues of the day is concerned with the selection of the particular social pattern through which the blessings of these medical advances shall be distributed among our people. For this reason, a discussion of the economics of medical care is timely; and only a fully informed public can arrive at a wise decision.

I am indebted to a number of friends for much assistance in the preparation of these lectures. Dr. Dwight E. Harken, of Harvard University, has graciously consented to give the greater part of the lecture upon the surgery of the heart and lungs, illustrated with his own incomparable motion pictures, in color, of actual operations. Doctor Harken was one of my valued associates in the medical service of the European Theater of Operations in the late war. This, his latest assistance to me, increases the heavy debt I already owe him.

To my old friend and comrade in arms, Brigadier General Raymond O. Dart, Director of the Army Institute of Pathology, I am indebted for the preparation of the lantern slides with which many of these lectures are illustrated; and to another fellow soldier, Colonel Joseph H. McNinch of the Army Medical Library, I owe thanks for the mass of reference material furnished me.

To my Secretary, Miss Lydia Wright, I am indebted for many tiresome hours spent in the library as well as in tedious revisions of the many drafts of the manuscripts of these lectures.

PAUL R. HAWLEY

Chicago
1 May 1949

CONTENTS

ILLUSTRATIONS

NEW DISCOVERIES
IN MEDICINE

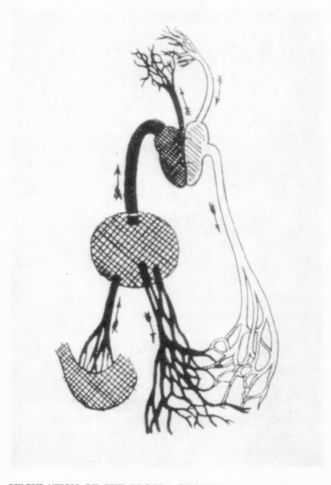

CIRCULATION OF THE BLOOD ACCORDING TO GALEN.

From *A History of Medicine,* by Artruro Castiglioni, 1941;
with permission of Alfred A. Knopf, Inc., Publishers.

OUR FABULOUS BLOOD

PART I

Ancient speculations and superstitions associated with blood. Early efforts at transmitting traits of character and personality through ingestion or transfusion of blood. Discovery of blood types and the impetus this gave to the development of transfusion. Importance of transfusion of blood and blood substitutes in the saving of life

MANY MORE IMPORTANT discoveries have been made in the field of the healing arts in the past twenty-five years than in any previous century of medical history. There has been during this period a great reduction in general mortality and in the case fatality of many diseases and injuries. Had the world been at peace throughout these years, the amazing effectiveness of the sulfonamides and the antibiotics might have obscured the importance of other great contributions toward the saving of life and the improvement of health.

But the concentration, rarely seen in peace, of severe injuries during war—the sudden mutilation of thousands of strong, healthy people—has recently focused attention upon equally dramatic lifesaving procedures. Among those not killed outright, hemorrhage and surgical shock have always been the principle causes of death from injuries. If only these two dangers could be survived, more often than not Nature made at least such repairs as were essential to life.

The most effective agent in combating surgical shock, and in counteracting the ill effects of the loss of blood, is blood itself. Especially as regards its effectiveness in hemorrhage, this would appear so obvious that it seems at first glance surprising that blood transfusion is but a recently developed technique in medicine and surgery. The fact is that the transfusion of blood from one person to another has long been a subject both of speculation and experimentation; but the chemical and biological complexity of blood was an obstacle that baffled investigators for centuries. Even now, after millions of hours of research and with blood transfusion an established procedure, there are some reactions in blood that are not well understood, and there may be others not yet suspected.

The value of blood as a restorative, and in the maintenance of health, is by no means limited to its role as a carrier of oxygen to the tissues of the body and as a remover of waste products therefrom. With the exception of only three or four specific and semispecific remedies, such as mercury and arsenic in syphilis and quinine in malaria, blood was the only specific curative agent known to medicine until the discovery of the sulfa drugs; and the range of its curative powers is far greater than that of any other remedy. The reason for this lies in the peculiar power of blood to develop its own unique and original compounds to combat specific organisms of disease with which it is brought into contact. Thus, blood is a living, flexible, and adaptable remedy without the limitations of fixed chemical compounds.

This property of blood has long been exploited in the development of antitoxins and other serums for the treatment of numerous diseases. But you must remember that your own blood will do as much as, and often more than, the blood of another animal injected into your body in the form of an antitoxin or other serum—provided only that you survive the onslaught of the disease long enough for your blood to get into full production. It usually requires considerable time for blood to develop such specific curative agents in adequate quantities, and the disease often progresses faster than the cure. It is safe to say that, with a few notable exceptions, our own blood would eventually cure all infections to which we are subject, provided only we survive the disease long enough for the blood to perfect a defense. Survival depends upon the ability of the blood to manufacture protective substances at a rate as fast or faster than the organisms of disease can manufacture lethal poisons. It is in this question of initial survival that the danger lies; and this is the reason for the constant search for specific remedies which will act more rapidly than blood.

The circulatory system has excited the curiosity of man for thousands of years. No other anatomical system—not even the nervous system with its mysterious brain—has provoked so much speculation; and around no other has been woven so many curious fantasies about the phenomena of life. At one time, all the vital forces were thought to be located in or controlled by the heart. Aristotle taught that the heart is the central abode of life, of the mind, and of the soul, the hearth from which generative animal heat emanates. In Biblical times, the processes of thought were believed to be centered in the heart. "As he thinketh in his own heart, so he is." [1] "So teach us to number our own days that we may apply our hearts unto wisdom." [2] "And immediately when Jesus perceived in his spirit that they so reasoned within themselves, He said unto them, Why

[1] Proverbs 23:7.　　　　　　　[2] Psalm XC, 12.

reason ye these things in your hearts?" [3] That this was a belief, and not merely a romantic figure of speech, is evidenced by the fact that Galen offered proof that it is not true. Basing his statement upon his observations of wounded gladiators, he reported that, "if a ventricle [of the heart] were wounded, these gladiators died very soon, and especially so if the left ventricle were wounded. If it was a nonpenetrating wound, they sometimes lived until the following day; and, as long as they lived, they were of the same mind, which is testimony that the heart is not the seat of the mind."

The attributes of character were located in the heart—brave heart, faint heart, hard heart, soft heart; men were chicken-hearted or lion-hearted. Jeremiah lamented that "The heart is deceitful above all things, and desperately wicked: Who can know it?" [4]

All human emotions were thought to center in the heart—love, hate, compassion, sorrow. "The heart bowed down by weight of woe." [5] "The heart can ne'er a transport know, That never feels a pain." [6] "And thus the heart will break, yet brokenly live on." [7]

It is not odd that primitive man's interest in himself focused his attention upon the heart. Denied accurate knowledge of internal anatomy by prohibitions against dissection of human bodies, his observations were largely limited to the surface of his body; and his concepts of physiology were thereby confined to highly speculative theories which were for the most part fallacious. The heart

[3] Mark 2:8.
[4] Jeremiah 17:9.
[5] Bunn, *Bohemian Girl.*
[6] Lyttleton, "Song."
[7] Byron, *Childe Harold's Pilgrimage.*

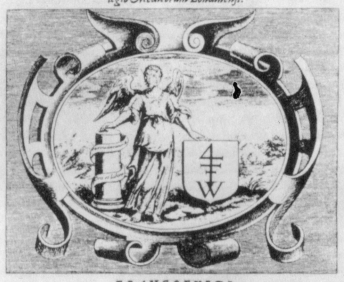

EXERCITATIO
ANATOMICA DE
MOTV CORDIS ET SAN-
GVINIS IN ANIMALI-
BVS,

GVILIELMI HARVEI ANGLI,
Medici Regii, & Profefforis Anatomiæ in Col-
legio Medicorum Londinenfi.

FRANCOFVRTI,
Sumptibus GVILIELMI FITZERI.

ANNO M. DC. XXVIII.

FIG. 1. FRONTISPIECE OF HARVEY'S EPOCH-MAKING PUBLICATION AN-
NOUNCING HIS DISCOVERY OF THE CIRCULATION OF THE BLOOD.

From *Cardiac Classics*, by F. A. Willius and T. E. Keys, eds., 1941; with
permission of the C. V. Mosby Company, Publishers.

was one of the larger viscera, and almost the only one whose presence was detectable by palpation. It was the only viscus which gave evidence of life perceivable to the unaided senses. It was in constant motion—hence a living organ. Furthermore, primitive man was not long in associating cardiac or precordial sensation with his emotional state. Sadness gave him a feeling of weight around his heart —hence a heavy heart—and, if intense and persistent, a broken heart. Fear provoked a "gone" feeling in the epigastrium, and perhaps with some air hunger—hence a faint heart. These and other emotions often produced palpitation of his heart, which made him acutely aware of its existence. And finally, his experience, both with his fellow men and with slaughtered animals, taught him that, when the heart ceased to live and to move, all life had ended. So his prepossession with the importance of his heart in all of his vital functions is easily understood.

Man, for many thousands of years, has entertained extraordinary ideas about blood. He has worshipped it, he has been terrified of it. He has accredited it with miraculous powers. Millions of human beings, not to speak of billions of animals, have been slaughtered that their blood might propitiate unfriendly gods. Blood sacrifice was a most important rite in the religion of the Old Testament; and today the technique of bleeding an animal or a fowl is an essential element of kosher slaughtering. In their human sacrifices, the ancient Aztecs plucked the living heart from the body of the victim, and offered it to their gods.

Aristotle held that both the blood and the blood vessels are derived from the heart. Since the heart remained approximately in its fixed location, the only obvious medium through which its many mystical powers could be trans-

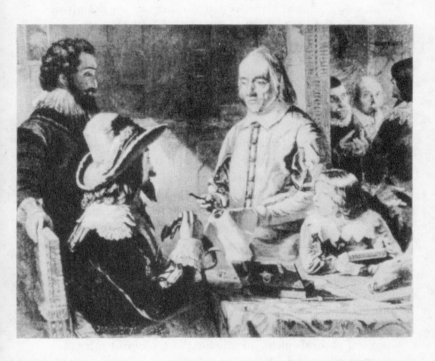

FIG. 2. WILLIAM HARVEY EXPOUNDING HIS CONCEPTION OF THE CIRCU-
LATION OF THE BLOOD TO KING CHARLES I OF ENGLAND.

From *Cardiac Classics*, by F. A. Willius and T. E. Keys, eds., 1941; with
permission of the C. V. Mosby Company, Publishers.

mitted to the rest of the body was the blood. Until about the beginning of the Christian era it was believed that only the veins carried blood, and that the arteries carried air. This was a natural error in that arteries are almost always found free of blood in the cadavers of both men and animals, for the reason that, during *rigor mortis,* in common with other muscles, the muscular walls of the arteries go into spasm and squeeze all of the blood into the veins. After *rigor mortis* has passed, the arterial walls relax, and the arteries then appear as hollow tubes containing only air.

After the distinction was made between arterial and venous blood, for thousands of years these two types of blood were considered as distinct entities. In the second century, Galen evolved his hypothesis upon the dynamics and the physiology of the blood. He originated the dogma that the blood ebbed and flowed with the beat of the heart, but did not circulate from the heart through the arteries and back to the heart through the veins. He taught that the arterial blood carries vital spirits from the heart—conforming with the traditional concept that the heart is the center of all life—and that the venous blood carries natural spirits from the liver. It is interesting to note in passing that relatively recent researches into liver function confirm Galen's idea—if "natural spirits" are defined as biological substances exerting profound effects upon other parts of the body. Galen's hypotheses were not fully satisfied in the absence of communication between the blood in the arteries and that in the veins; and, to supply this deficiency, Galen invented invisible pores through the septum separating the ventricles of the heart, and through which, he said, there is communication between the arterial blood in the left ventricle and the venous blood in the right ventricle.

Galen's views were accepted practically without question throughout Europe for almost 1400 years. Obviously, during these 14 centuries there was little medical investigation worthy of the name. Such pseudoscientific dogmas as those of Galen became cloaked with religious sanctity. Observations in conflict with them were discredited—often by the observers themselves. So, when William Harvey announced, in 1616, his discovery of the circulation of the blood, he was attacked upon all sides as a medical antichrist—an unscrupulous iconoclast who dared question the established wisdom of the ages.

While Harvey's discovery settled many questions of the dynamics of blood, it added nothing to the knowledge of its chemistry and histology, and little to the understanding of its physiology. Blood played a very important part in the earlier concepts of genetics—and still does in many lay minds. Inherited characteristics were thought to repose in the blood. People came of good blood, or of bad blood. Curiously enough, the aristocracy were blue-blooded people, perhaps because the blue veins were more visible through a skin not toughened and tanned by toil and by exposure to the elements. The transmission of characteristics through the medium of blood was also believed possible outside the generative process. With the idea of assimilating desirable qualities, primitive peoples drank the blood of ferocious animals, and savages gorged upon the blood of slain enemies who had displayed commendable courage. Even today, butchers will extol the value of fresh, warm blood as a builder of health and strength.

The influence of the state of the blood upon disease and upon health has been expounded in many printed pages; and some of the old superstitions are still in circulation.

Blood became too thick in the winter, and had to be thinned each spring, either by venesection or by vile potions concocted from herbs. Physicians bled their patients for every indisposition, mild or grave—a practice that has persisted to this day, with the symbolic substitution of the purse for the vein.

The pioneering work of Harvey did much more for biological science than to add one fact, however startling, to the sum of knowledge about the human body. It opened eyes to the weaknesses in the foundation upon which had been erected a fantastic structure of theories of anatomy and physiology. Once released from the bondage imposed by Galen and other ancients, men with curious minds set about searching for facts to substitute for existing fancies. Harvey was scarcely dead before experimenters in England and on the Continent were trying to transfuse the blood of one animal into the vessels of another—of the same or different species.[8] This was before the discovery of the cellular elements of blood in man, although the red blood cells had been observed by Schwammerdam, in a frog, a few years before.

It is interesting to speculate upon the objective of these early experimenters in transfusion. Since nothing was then known of blood volume and blood pressure, and their relation to surgical shock, nor of the oxygen-carrying capacity of blood and its essentiality to life, one must conjecture that at least one of the things they had in mind was the transmission of personal characteristics. The view of the day

[8] These experiments were, however, not the first effort at transfusion. Transfusion, as a therapeutic procedure, had been considered for two or three hundred years. It is possible that Pope Innocent VIII was transfused in the fifteenth century.

admitted to the possibility of gentling a ferocious lion by transfusing him with the blood of a sheep. It may be that some of these early investigators, caught in a turbulent domestic situation, were searching for a scientific method of taming a shrew. On the other hand, it is quite possible that the experimenters had a no better-defined objective than merely to see what would happen—a type of investigation which has made some amazing contributions to the sum of human knowledge.

Insofar as the early London experiments are concerned, Samuel Pepys supports my contention that the primary objective was to demonstrate whether or not characteristics of temperament could be transmitted through blood transfusion, and whether the practice might not be useful in the treatment of disease by substituting good blood for bad. Pepys, for some reason, missed the first demonstration at the Royal Society; but he was told of the results within a few hours, and he commented in this vein: "This did give rise to many pretty wishes, as of the blood of a Quaker to be let into an Archbishop and such like; but, as Dr. Croone says, may if it takes be of mighty use to man's health, for the amending of bad blood by borrowing from a better body."

In the first Royal Society experiment, an artery of a small mastiff dog was in some way connected with a vein of a spaniel, probably through the use of a silver, or other metallic, tube. Another distant blood vessel of the spaniel was opened, so that the latter's own blood drained to waste as it was replaced by the blood of the mastiff. The mastiff, of course, bled to death; but, two days later, Pepys noted in his diary that he had learned that "the dog which was filled with another's dog's blood, at the College the other day, is very well and like to be so as ever;" and his informant went on to say that he "doubts not [this demonstration] being found of great use to men." Pepys added that this view also was taken by his friend, Dr. Whistler.

I should like to digress for a moment to observe that, to too many people, Samuel Pepys was but a naughty little man who recorded his peccadilloes in a diary of which, until quite recently, only expurgated editions have been available. His famous diary gives a highly erroneous picture of the man. Actually, he was one of the ablest men of his generation; and his contribution to the development of the British Navy has exerted a profound influence upon the history of the world until our own day. To those who really want to know Samuel Pepys, I commend Arthur Bryant's three-volume biography.

The success of this first experiment encouraged the investigators to plan a bolder step at once. They found a human subject who was agreeable, for a consideration of twenty shillings, to receiving a transfusion of blood from a sheep. This volunteer human guinea pig was obviously ignorant of the potentialities of the procedure—as, of course, were the experimenters themselves—rather than either courageous or a willing martyr to science. Pepys describes him as being by nature "a little frantic"—whatever he meant by that—"a kind of a minister [of the Gospel], that is a poor and debauched man." In any event, the frantic little man was given, by direct transfusion, what was estimated to be about twelve ounces of sheep's blood. Pepys saw him six days later, and stated that "he speaks well and did this day give the Society a relation [of his experience] in Latin, saying that he finds himself much better since, and is a new man; but he is cracked a little in his head, though he speaks very reasonably and very well." Pepys went on to say that a repetition of the experiment upon the same subject was planned, but he did not again mention it in his diary. Actually, the experiment was repeated upon this subject, but the results were so inconclusive that they were never published in the Transactions of the Royal Society. The amount of sheep's blood transfused into this man may have been too small to have caused any serious consequences upon the first occasion. But it was probably enough to have sensitized him against sheep's blood, so that the second transfusion would have produced a reaction that might well have proved fatal, had any great amount of sheep's blood reached the man's circulation.

After these seventeenth century experiments, interest in blood transfusion waned, probably for two reasons. First, the procedure was found to be dangerous, and the causes of severe reactions were obscure; and, second, the original purposes could not be shown to be valid. It was not until the field of surgery was greatly extended through the discoveries of anesthesia and aseptic techniques that a real demand for blood transfusion was created.

When these early experiments in transfusion were made, little was known of the constitution of the blood. It was regarded as a homogeneous solution. The discovery of the cellular elements of the blood awaited the development of the compound microscope, since the power of the simple magnifying glass was too low to reveal them. Blood corpuscles were first identified as such by Antony van Leeuwenhoek in 1674. But more than two hundred years were to elapse before the existence of the immunological phenomena in blood was even suspected.

The interest of investigators in the possibility of transfusing blood from one person to another was revived around the turn of the present century. The frequent reactions, often severe and occasionally fatal, pointed to some source or sources of incompatibility of the bloods of two individuals. The first step in the solution of this problem of incompatibility was made by Karl Landsteiner in 1900, when he discovered the existence of three blood types; and further study soon added a fourth type.

Actually, the four types are the result of combinations of only two factors of incompatibility. This is perhaps best illustrated by the accompanying table.

Blood Types, and the Sources of Incompatibility among Them

Blood Type	Red Blood Cell Antigens Present	Blood Serum Antibodies Present	Per cent of White People * with This Type
A	A	anti-B	40.4
B	B	anti-A	11.6
AB	A and B	none	7.5
O	none	anti-A and anti-B	40.6

* The incidence varies among different races.

At this point it may prove helpful to digress briefly to explain the more essential elements of an antigen-antibody reaction. One of the characteristics of blood is that, when certain types of foreign substances, known as antigens, are introduced into it, the blood reacts to form biochemical products which will neutralize or destroy the foreign substances. Antigens are practically always wholly protein, or contain a protein fraction. So, when a red cell containing Type A antigen is exposed to blood serum containing antibodies against Type A antigen, that cell is destroyed.

The usual method of destruction of red cells by antagon-

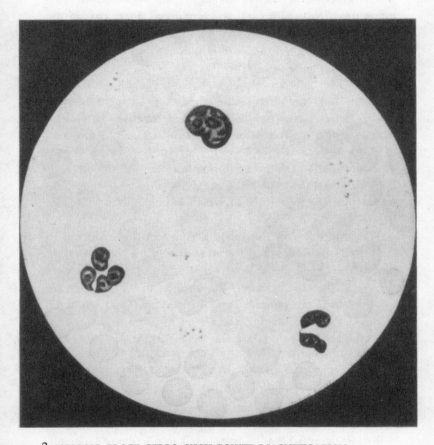

FIG. 3. NORMAL BLOOD CELLS; HIGH-POWER MAGNIFICATION.

From *Color Atlas of Hematology*, by R. R. Kracke, 1947; with permission of the J. B. Lippincott Company, Publishers.

istic antibodies is one of agglutination followed by disintegration. Normally each red blood cell floats free in the blood serum. This is necessary for their passage through the tiny capillaries, the lumens of which are only a little larger than the diameter of a red cell.

When red cells are attacked by antagonistic antibodies, the first thing that happens is that their surfaces become sticky. This causes red cells to stick together in clumps instead of floating free as individual cells. This phenomenon of clumping, whether of blood cells or of bacteria, is known as agglutination. After agglutination the red blood cells begin to die. Eventually they burst and discharge their contents, the most important of which is hemoglobin, into the blood serum.

The antibodies in the blood serum are the evildoers in the reactions following the transfusion of incompatible blood. They are specific agents that agglutinate and destroy the red cells which contain the antigen to which they are antagonistic. For example, Type A blood has Type A antigen in the red cells. However, the serum of Type A blood contains no antibodies against this type of antigen—otherwise this blood would destroy its own red cells. So, Type A blood can be injected into a person who has Type A blood without danger from this cause, since there are no antibodies against Type A antigen in the blood of either the donor or recipient.

But, if Type B blood is transfused into a Type A person, the anti-B antibodies in the blood serum of the recipient set about immediately to destroy the red blood cells of the donor which contain B antigen. A similar phenomenon occurs if Type A blood is injected into the blood stream of a Type B person.

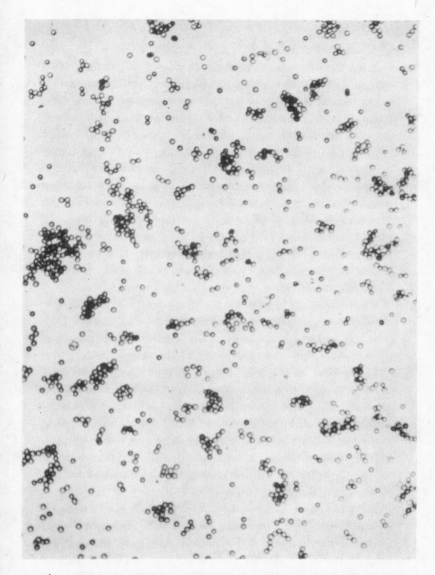

FIG. 4. AGGLUTINATION OF BLOOD; LOW-POWER MAGNIFICATION. NOTE
THE CLUMPING OF THE RED CELLS.

From *Rh*, by Edith L. Potter, 1947; with permission of the Year Book
Publishers.

Type AB people are known as "universal recipients." This means that any other type of blood—A, B, or O—may be given them without reaction from incompatibility. The reason for this is obvious; the serum of Type AB people contains no antibodies against such antigens, and consequently neither A nor B antigen is attacked by the serum of a Type AB person.

Conversely, Type O people are known as "universal donors," since their red cells contain no antigen to be attacked by Anti-A or Anti-B antibodies. Only Type O blood was supplied to the armed forces overseas during the late war because this simplified the distribution of bottled whole blood—only one type having to be stocked instead of four—and made typing of recipents unnecessary.

I am sure that already one big question has arisen in your minds: If Type O blood contains antibodies against both A and B antigen, how can it be universally used? Why does it not destroy the red blood cells of the recipient?

The answer to this lies in the fact that the donor's blood is added slowly to the blood of the recipient, and is diluted almost immediately upon its entrance into the recipient's vein. On the other hand, the red cells of the donor's blood immediately encounter a heavy concentration of antibodies in the recipient's blood, and are agglutinated at once if antagonistic antibodies are present in the blood of the recipient. Furthermore, ordinarily the amount of donor's blood given is much smaller than the volume of the recipient's blood. So, the reaction following the transfusion of incompatible blood is due almost entirely to the destruction of the red cells of the donor by the serum of the recipient, rather than either to the opposite reaction or to mutual destruction.

The complete cause of reactions following transfusions

of incompatible blood are not yet known. It is known that the products of the disintegration of red blood cells are toxic. Particularly is this true of hemoglobin. Free hemoglobin in the blood serum produces profound symptoms. If sufficient in amount it totally blocks the tubules of the kidneys, and death results from uremia. The suspension of kidney function from this blockage of tubules is the most common cause of death following the transfusion of incompatible blood.

The discovery of the blood types has had a much wider application than in the prevention of reactions following blood transfusion. It is applied every day to the partial identification of the source of blood in criminal cases. Fortunately, the type of blood can be determined from old, dried blood stains—even if they must be scraped from objects. If the type of blood found in spots upon a suspect's clothing is different from that of his own blood but the same as that of the blood of the injured or murdered person, it is not conclusive evidence that the blood stains were made by the victim's blood, but it adds to the chain of circumstances that point to the guilt of the suspect. On the other hand, if the blood type of the stain is different from that of the victim, it is certain that the stain was not made by the victim's blood.

Since there are only the four types of blood, the evidence adduced from comparing blood types can only be conclusive when it is negative. When two bloods match in type, it may be coincidence. They may be the same blood, or they may be the bloods of two different people of the same blood type.

Blood type is a Mendelian characteristic. For this reason it has assumed some importance in establishing the parentage of offspring of disputed descent. Combinations of parents of certain blood types can produce offspring only of certain types. In the accompanying table are shown all the possible hereditary combinations of blood types.

Thus, if the blood of the child was A, and that of the mother was O the father must have been of Type A or Type

Possible Hereditary Combinations of Blood Types

Blood Groups of Parents	Possible Blood Groups of Children
O and O	O
O and A	O or A
O and B	O or B
A and A	O or A
A and B	O, A, B, or AB
B and B	O or B
O and AB	A or B
A and AB	A, B, or AB
B and AB	A, B, or AB
AB and AB	A, B, or AB

AB. If the blood of the suspected father is of Type B or Type O, he must be cleared of all complicity. If the blood type of both mother and child is O, then the father must also be of Type O. No man with blood of type A, B, or AB, can father a child of Type O by a mother of Type O.

You will note that the value of this test varies with the combinations of blood types of parents. When one parent is of Type A and the other of Type B, the test is worthless in the establishment of relationship, because of the fact the offspring can be of any of the four blood types. Also, here again, an agreement is not evidence—it is only a possibility; but a disagreement is conclusive evidence. Type O parents can have an O-type offspring—but they can be any two O-type persons of different sexes. But two Type O parents can never have offspring of A, B, or AB-type blood.

PART II

*Development of blood transfusion as a therapeutic technique.
The whole blood and plasma program of World War II,
and its influence upon the saving of battle casualties. Modern blood banks and the Red Cross Blood Bank Program*

W<small>E</small> <small>HAVE NOTED</small> that the possibility of transfusing the
blood of an animal, including man, into the circulation of
another individual of the same or different species had excited curiosity for at least three hundred years, and probably longer. One author of the sixteenth century published
a pamphlet in which he described, with the assistance of
detailed drawings, an apparatus for blood transfusion. The
importance of his contribution was lessened, however, by
his frank statement that he had never tested his invention.

The early experimenters became discouraged both by the
physical and mechanical difficulties not easily overcome by
crude apparatuses, and by resultant phenomena beyond
their comprehension. The frequency of severe and even
fatal reactions following the mixture of incompatible bloods
leads one to believe that the pioneers in the field were not
so successful as their published reports might indicate.

It was many years after the anatomy and physiology of
the blood was fairly well understood that its immunologic
reactions began to be suspected. The new science of bac-
teriology, born late in the nineteenth century, first revealed
the existence of such phenomena; and it was therefore
natural that early immunologists concerned themselves almost exclusively with the reaction of blood to the invasion
of bacteria. It was not long, however, before a few curious

investigators widened their interest in the study of the reaction of blood to all foreign substances, including admixtures of different bloods. They found that such reactions were, for the most part, comparable with the bacteria-antibody reactions first discovered; and this general class of phenomena is now known as antigen-antibody reactions.

It was Landsteiner who first reported the presence of specific antigens in the red blood cells of some people and their absence in others, and also the presence or absence of antibodies in the blood serum of people which attacked these antigens. On the basis of his discovery, it was found that the blood of human beings can be classified into four general types—A, B, AB, and O. There are varying degrees of incompatibility among these types, and much depends upon whether an individual be a donor or a recipient in a blood transfusion. The only completely safe transfusion is one in which the blood of the donor is of the same type as that of the recipient, although, in practice, O-type persons are regarded as universal donors and AB-type persons as universal recipients.

For a number of years after Landsteiner's work was reported, clinicians believed that most of the problems of blood transfusion had been solved. Occasional reactions—some severe and occasionally a fatal one—were still experienced; but these were usually explained upon the ground of contamination of the donor's blood with some foreign substance. It was known that there is such a class of foreign substances, generically termed pyrogens, which cannot be detected and cannot be excluded from glassware and tubing by ordinary methods of cleaning and sterilization; and these post-transfusion reactions with typed bloods were usually ascribed to pyrogens.

But hematologists were not satisfied with such a plausible explanation. They continued inquiries into the immunology and biochemistry of blood; and their efforts have recently been rewarded by the discovery of individual variations in blood other than those classified by Landsteiner *et al.* One of these is the Rh factor. There are still others; and recently there was reported in the public press the discovery of a special type of antigen which appears thus far to be found only in the members of one family.

As the result of the work by Landsteiner and others, the practice of blood transfusion, on other than an experimental scale, began to increase around 1907. The first technique was one of actual joining of an artery of the donor to a vein of the recipient—vessels in the forearms of each being generally used. This was a tedious procedure, not without danger to both donor and recipient. It required skilled surgery, and the sacrifice of an artery of the donor as well as a vein of the recipient. Neither vessel could again be used for transfusion. A further source of danger, which limited the usefulness of the procedure, especially in children and in other patients not fully conscious or rational, was that movement on the part of one or the other parties involved might sever the temporary connection between the vessels and ruin the operation. This type of transfusion is known as direct transfusion.

The next few years saw the development of many types of apparatuses designed to avoid the necessity for sewing the artery of the donor to the vein of the recipient. The common principle of all of these was the substitution of hollow needles and tubing for the direct connection of the artery and vein. In some, the arterial pressure of the donor was depended upon for the flow to the recipient; and, in other types, a pump and reservoir both augmented the rate of flow and permitted measurement of the amount of blood transfused. The great difficulty with this type of procedure is in the prevention of the coagulation of the blood of the donor before it reaches the vein of the recipient.

Since rough surfaces favor coagulation of blood, many expedients were tried to remove this factor, such as coating the interiors of the tubing and glassware of the apparatuses with smooth substances like paraffin. None was entirely successful, and inability to prevent coagulation during transfusion precluded widespread use of the direct-indirect method of transfusion.

The inherent difficulties of the direct method of blood transfusion led Richard Lewisohn, of the staff of Mount Sinai Hospital in New York, in 1914, to search for a better method—one which would permit of a more leisurely technique whereby blood could be collected from a donor in one operation and administered to a recipient in another. The key to the solution of this problem, as Lewisohn recognized, lay in the prevention of the coagulation of the blood during the period in which it was outside the bodies of both donor and recipient.

Although the biochemistry of the coagulation of blood is a relatively recent discovery—and not yet fully understood —it has been known for almost a century that the addition of certain foreign substances will prevent the coagulation of blood. Perhaps the first observation of this nature was that blood does not coagulate in the digestive system of certain blood-sucking insects and other creatures. Leeches were used for many years to remove blood from people— both from the circulatory system in the treatment of systemic diseases and from contusions in which blood vessels

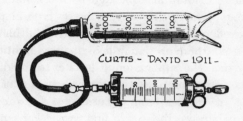

CURTIS · DAVID · 1911 ·

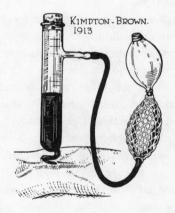

KIMPTON · BROWN.
1913

FIG. 5. APPARATUSES FOR TRANSFUSION OF UNMOD-
IFIED BLOOD USING PARAFFIN-LINED CONTAINERS.

From *The Blood Bank and the Technique and Ther-
apeutics of Transfusion*, by R. A. Kilduffe and M. E.
DeBakey, 1942; with permission of the C. V. Mosby
Company, Publishers.

had been ruptured and blood had escaped into the tissues to cause the discoloration associated with bruises. Less than a century ago, live leeches were a most important item of a well-stocked pharmacy; and even today, although they are rarely used, there are much less effective treatments for a black eye than the application of leeches to the discolored area. I have often speculated upon the reasons for the disappearance of leeches from pharmacies. I do not know whether it is because they were first replaced by raw beefsteak and later by cosmetics, or whether fewer people run into doors than did so formerly.

So, it was natural that, in his search for a suitable anticoagulant, Lewisohn turned first to the leech. The reason that blood does not coagulate in the digestive system of the leech is that there is secreted in the mouth of the leech a substance known as hirudin which, when mixed with fresh blood, prevents coagulation. Lewisohn first tried hirudin, but found it too toxic for use in human transfusions.

He then turned to chemical salts, of which several were already known to be anticoagulants. The first of these salts to be discovered were poisonous in the amounts required, and it was not until the discovery was made that sodium citrate was an adequate anticoagulant, and relatively harmless even in large doses, that the procedure of transfusion was freed both from serious technical difficulties and from much of its danger. A soluble calcium salt, a normal constituent of blood plasma, is an essential element in the formation of blood clot. The chemical anticoagulants merely inactivate the calcium ions and thus prevent coagulation. Thus, when sodium citrate is added to fresh blood, the calcium ions are fixed without precipitation, and the blood can no longer clot.

This discovery greatly accelerated the development of blood transfusion. Lewisohn and Baehr developed its use and transformed the procedure from a complicated, uncertain operation, with a considerable element of danger, to one of comparative simplicity relatively free from danger. No longer was it necessary for donor and recipient to be brought close together. Blood could be withdrawn from the donor into a flask containing a small amount of a solution of sodium citrate, and taken to the recipient in another part of the hospital. This is known as the indirect method of blood transfusion. A reasonable delay between the collection and the administration of the blood was permissible. However, the preservation of collected blood for days, rather than minutes, was a matter of later development; and, for some years, it was necessary to obtain an individual donor each time a transfusion was indicated.

During World War I the value of restoring the blood volume after severe hemorrhage was well recognized. However, the indirect method of transfusion, developed only after the start of the war and less than two years prior to the entry of the United States in this war, had not yet achieved wide acceptance and was not generally used. So, most of the transfusions were by the direct method with the use of one or another type of syringe or pump. But the difficulty of obtaining donors in sufficient numbers in the battle zone was so great that whole blood was used rather infrequently. Certainly, its use was upon a scale not to be compared with that of the late war. Instead, blood volume was most often restored by the injection of blood substitutes. Normal salt solution was first used; but this was retained in the circulation for such a short time that it was not a satisfactory blood substitute. Other substances, notably gum acacia, were added to the salt solution to increase its viscosity and thus retard its excretion. These thicker solutions were improvements, but the results fell far short of the results obtained with whole blood.

The surgeons of that day—and, for that matter, the surgeons to the time of World War II—seem to have regarded the restoration of blood volume and of blood pressure to be about all that is required in surgical shock unless the patient be almost wholly exsanguinated. Since cases of anemia do reasonably well at rest with less than half the normal amount of red blood cells, the loss of oxygen-carrying capacity after severe hemorrhage seems not to have impressed medical men.

It is true that oxygen is soluble in the plasma of the blood, but only mildly so. If there were no red cells in the blood, a circulating volume 75 times as great as normal would be required to carry the same amount of oxygen as is carried by red cells. Each gram of hemoglobin in the red cells of the blood will carry 1.34 cc. of oxygen, so that normal blood fully oxygenated contains 20 percent of oxygen. Without the hemoglobin, blood could absorb only a little more than one-fourth of one percent of oxygen.

For this reason, all blood substitutes, including blood plasma, are practically worthless as oxygen carriers, and their usefulness is limited to building the blood volume so that the vessels are better filled and the blood pressure is brought back toward normal. The maintenance of adequate blood pressure is essential to the action of the heart. If blood pressure falls below a critical point, which varies slightly in different people, the heart stops.

Unquestionably, the difficulties encountered in preserving whole blood longer than a very few hours retarded the early development of its use. The cellular elements are the most fragile and most perishable. When separated from the blood cells, blood plasma, even in its natural, liquid state, keeps well when stored in a refrigerator. But the blood cells tend to disintegrate when whole blood is stored, and the red cells burst and liberate hemoglobin into the

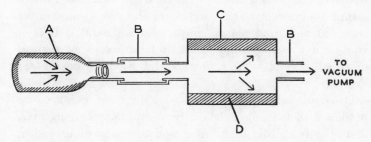

FIG. 6. SCHEMATIC REPRESENTATION OF ESSENTIAL COMPO-
NENTS OF ANY PLASMA-DRYING SYSTEM. A: SHELL OF FROZEN
PLASMA. B: CONNECTING TUBE. C: CONDENSER. D: WATER
CONDENSATE, EITHER FROZEN ON A COLD SURFACE OR AB-
SORBED BY A CHEMICAL DESICCATE.

From *Blood Derivatives and Substitutes*, by C. S. White and J. J.
Weinstein, 1947; with permission of the Williams and Wilkins
Company, Publishers.

plasma. This is known as hemolysis of the blood. Hemo-lyzed blood cannot be used in transfusion. It causes very serious and often fatal reactions. The white cells are even more perishable and disappear from stored blood within six to twenty-four hours. However, a bit of research has just now been reported in which a method of preserving white blood cells has been discovered. This will extend the field of usefulness of transfused blood.

Between the World Wars, a method of drying blood

plasma was developed whereby the water is removed, leaving the solids—the blood proteins and the salts—in a powdered, crystalline form. This dried plasma will keep indefinitely, and its value, particularly in war, was recognized at once. It became possible to collect blood in enormous amounts from thousands of donors, to separate the plasma from the cells, and to dry and store the plasma against future emergencies. The addition of the proper amount of water to the dried plasma reconstitutes it, and it is then ready for injection. Thousands and thousands of pounds of dried plasma were prepared and used during World War II.

Dried plasma has the great advantages of being easily prepared, of keeping indefinitely at ordinary temperatures, and of being easily distributed and easily administered in the battle zone—even at the very front lines. It has the disadvantages, however, of being much less effective than whole blood, and of being a carrier of at least one virus infection—that of infectious jaundice.

Whole blood also may and does carry virus infections. But it is much simpler to process and store whole blood in individual lots—that is, the blood of only one donor in each bottle. To process dried plasma economically and practically, the blood plasma of hundreds of donors is pooled and dried as a whole. Thus the blood of only one carrier of a virus infection contaminates large stocks of dried plasma, and hundreds of recipients may be infected, whereas one bottle of whole blood infects only one recipient. Physical examination or other test will usually rule out communicable disease in a donor. However, otherwise healthy donors sometimes are carriers of a virus disease which cannot be detected by examination. The blood of

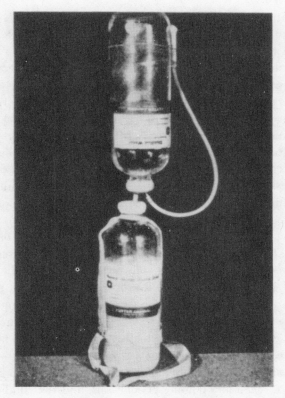

FIG. 7. RECONSTITUTION OF DRIED PLASMA. THE
STERILE DISTILLED WATER IS ADDED TO THE DRIED
PLASMA BY MEANS OF A STERILE DOUBLE-ENDED
NEEDLE. WHEN ALL WATER IS ADDED, AND THE
DRIED PLASMA IS DISSOLVED, IT IS READY FOR
ADMINISTRATION.

From *Blood Derivatives and Substitutes,* by C. S.
White and J. J. Weinstein, 1947; with permission of
the Williams and Wilkins Company, Publishers.

such donors transmits the disease to the recipients. Recently, methods of sterilizing plasma have been perfected, so that this danger has been eliminated.

The advantages of dried plasma were well known at the outset of World War II, and it was used on a large scale. The disadvantages were not so well recognized. Experience with badly wounded soldiers soon indicated that, in many cases, much more was necessary to save them than the mere restoration of their blood volume with reconstituted plasma. Replacement of lost oxygen-carrying power was found also to be essential. And soon, outbreaks of infectious jaundice, following transfusion with reconstituted plasma, pointed the danger from such unrecognizable contamination.

The United States was forced into World War II on the 7th of December, 1941. Early in 1942 we began to assemble our forces in Great Britain; and, during 1943 and the first half of 1944, our strength in Europe was built up in preparation for the invasion of the Continent. In these months of preparation our medical service was carefully studying British experience with blood substitutes, especially in the desert campaign. All this time we were suffering casualties in the air, but the number of our wounded was too small for us to reach any definite conclusions, and the conditions under which they were treated were quite different than those in which ground soldiers have to be treated. We did, however, suspect that we could, with benefit, use more whole blood and less plasma if it were possible for us to produce and distribute the whole blood. With this in mind, we organized our blood bank in the European Theater of Operations in the latter part of 1943. Our blood bank was in charge of Dr. Ralph Muckenfuss, of the New York City Department of Health, and a grand job he did with it. We

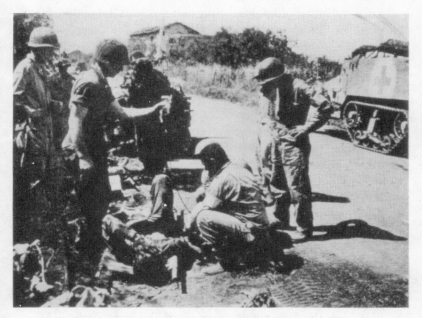

FIG. 8. TRANSFUSION OF A WOUNDED SOLDIER OF THE 1ST ARMORED
DIVISION WITH PLASMA DURING A BATTLE IN ITALY. THE EASE OF
ADMINISTRATION OF RECONSTITUTED PLASMA PERMITS OF ITS USE
UNDER ADVERSE CONDITIONS AT THE FRONT.

From *Blood Derivatives and Substitutes*, by C. S. White and J. J. Wein-
tein, 1947; with permission of the Williams and Wilkins Company, Publishers.

were furnished all the dried plasma from the United States
that we could use; so our only concern was a source of
whole blood. At that time it seemed, from British experience and after adding a wide margin for safety, that 500
pints of blood per day would be ample for our forces.
Whereas, in the desert campaign, the British had used four
or five pints of plasma to each pint of whole blood, we
estimated on the basis of two pints of plasma to each pint
of blood.

During the first week of the invasion of France, the demand for whole blood was very heavy. Our forward hospitals on the Normandy beaches were using one pint of
whole blood for each pint of plasma, instead of the one to
two ratio we had estimated. It was evident that we could
not long supply such a large amount of whole blood; and
I hastened to the front to stop what appeared to be unnecessary use of whole blood when plasma would have suf-
ficed. It took only a few hours, and an examination of
several hundred severely wounded men, to convince me
that whole blood was infinitely superior to plasma in all
but slightly injured patients. It was impossible to use whole
blood on the firing line, because of the care with which
stocks of blood must be handled, and plasma ordinarily
would support the severely wounded until they could reach
a forward hospital a few miles behind the line. But once
they reached the hospital and required emergency surgery,
only whole blood would restore and support them.

I flew back to England and started to expand our own
blood bank there. It was apparent, however, that our maximum capacity would never be more than 750 pints per day.
Since the British were bleeding their civil population for
their own military needs, for our own source of blood we

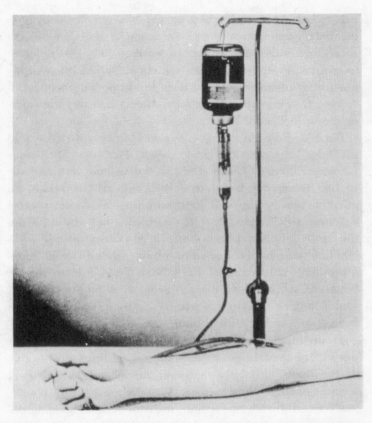

FIG. 9. TRANSFUSION WITH PRESERVED WHOLE BLOOD, SHOWING
THE METHOD OF HANGING THE BOTTLE OF BLOOD, THE FILTER
DRIP (TO MEASURE THE RATE OF ADMINISTRATION), THE
SHUT-OFF CLAMP, AND THE NEEDLE IN THE VEIN. PLASMA
MAY ALSO BE ADMINISTERED IN THIS WAY.

From *Blood Derivatives and Substitutes*, by C. S. White and J. J.
Weinstein, 1947; with permission of the Williams and Wilkins
Company, Publishers.

had to rely upon our service troops in rear areas and upon combat divisions awaiting the crossing of the Channel. As more and more of our troops entered the battle, there would be fewer from which we could get blood; and, as our forces advanced, supply lines would be lengthened and service troops scattered thereby—thus increasing the difficulties in collecting blood.

But blood we had to have, or many American lads would die who otherwise could be saved. So I sent Brigadier General Elliott C. Cutler back to the United States by air to beg for whole blood from this side of the ocean. So effective was his mission that, within a couple of months, we were receiving 1,000 pints of blood daily by air from the United States. Large 4-engine airplanes, loaded with whole blood, landed in Britain often in less than 20 hours after they had taken off from New York. I have seen a bottle of whole blood being given to a badly wounded soldier in Germany in less than 96 hours after it was taken from a vein in the United States.

To my mind, the distribution of whole blood at the front during the months of heavy fighting in Europe was one of the finest of all the accomplishments of the medical service of that theater. One of our refrigerator trucks, loaded with blood, was ashore in Normandy as soon as the first wave of our troops had cleared the beaches. The beaches were still under a perfect storm of fire; but the resourceful driver of this truck prevailed upon an engineer soldier to scoop out an enormous fox hole with a bulldozer; and he drove the blood truck into this excavation, remaining there for several days until a safer blood bank could be established elsewhere in the beachhead. From this buried truck, jeeps delivered blood to the evacuation and field

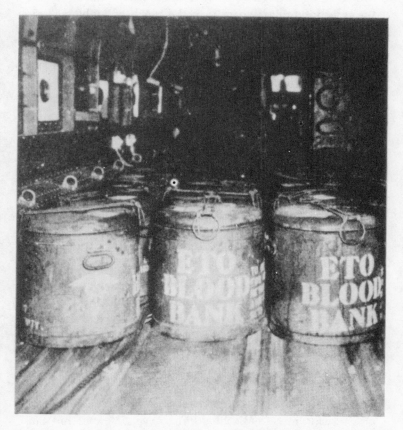

FIG. 10. A C-47 TRANSPORT PLANE LOADED WITH WHOLE BLOOD FROM THE EUROPEAN THEATER OF OPERATIONS BLOOD BANK, FOR DELIVERY TO FORWARD DISTRIBUTING POINTS.

From the *Military Surgeon*, July 1948; with permission of the Editor.

hospitals, operating twenty-four hours a day and scurrying through unfamiliar territory in the black of night with no lights to help. These young officers and men who manned the forward echelon of blood distribution did a magnificent job; and to their devoted and tireless efforts many an American soldier owes his life.

Blood is too perishable to be entrusted to slow transport. As our armies advanced into France, and distances became too great for economical use of motor transport, forward banks were established near the front lines, and these forward banks were supplied by air. This assured the freshness of the blood supplies to the front. While the storage life of whole blood is usually placed at 14 to 15 days, it was rare that blood as old as 10 days was used, and the average age of blood used in the most forward of our hospitals was only 6 to 8 days. Due to the fine processing and careful handling en route, only an insignificant amount spoiled. When it is considered that bottled blood must be kept at a constant low temperature, that freezing will ruin it, and that rough handling will break up the red cells and render it useless and even dangerous, the splendid performance of the blood supply system becomes apparent. So essential did whole blood become that any serious shortage at the front would have been productive of screams of anguish on the part of surgeons that could have been heard all the way back to Washington. I never knew of but one instance in which a hospital ran out of whole blood. This was a forward hospital in a remote spot, and the shortage lasted only 12 hours during which sufficient blood was obtained "on the hoof"—an army expression for bleeding volunteer donors on the spot.

It has been my fortune, or misfortune, to have been

closely associated with wounded soldiers in two World Wars. In both wars the wounded were young Americans, but there the resemblance ended. In World War I, the typical wounded man was obviously sick—pale, thin, and burning with fever. The hospital ward, in which he lay, smelled of pus.

The wounded soldier of World War II looked as if he had just come in from a game of tennis or a swim. He was not sick, and he did not look sick. Even those with severe wounds, unless the digestive tract was involved, consumed large meals on full diets. They were hungry and they liked their food. The wards were free from odor, because there was little or no infection. This great difference was the result of plasma and whole blood, and of penicillin and the sulfonamides. Surely, military surgery—and all surgery, for that matter—advanced more in the twenty-five years between World Wars than it did in the previous three centuries.

The use of whole blood in the treatment of disease and injured would have increased had there been no World War II. But it would have increased much more slowly. More than 40,000 doctors in the armed forces during World War II had the opportunity of observing the almost miraculous restorative properties of transfused whole blood; and this experience greatly accelerated the demand for blood in the civil practice of medicine. Prior to the war, blood banks were relatively few in number, and they were unable to meet the postwar demand. To meet this expanded need, the American National Red Cross instituted its blood bank program shortly after the end of the war. This program has been developed rapidly under the direction of

Admiral Ross T. McIntire, who was the Surgeon General of the Navy before and during the war years. Already there are agencies in every large city in the country and many in smaller communities.

I know of no finer channel through which the individual can contribute to the welfare of his fellow man than through the donation of some of his blood to a blood bank. In so doing, he not only gives a part of himself, but he gives a part which may well mean the difference between life and death to a fellow creature. The donation of blood to a blood bank has the added virtue of anonymity, and the donor is spared a parading of his philanthropy. Furthermore, blood is a gift which costs the donor nothing but the time required for its withdrawal. The blood he gives is rapidly replaced, and the donor is none the poorer for his generosity.

It occurs to me that, like many another of man's blundering efforts to improve the world, he has been directing his search abroad for the cures of diseases which afflict him, whereas the most effective cures have all the while been within his own body. We may expect that the near future will bring not only an increased use of blood in the treatment of disease and injury, but also more careful search for methods of enhancing the value of blood, such as by stimulating the rapidity of its reaction to the invasion of our bodies by harmful substances.

I am reminded of the old proverb that "a prophet is not without honor save in his own country." From time immemorial, blood has been accorded a respect approaching that due divinity, but largely in fields foreign to the everyday life of the individual. Miraculous as have been the virtues attributed to blood, it is most miraculous as it goes quietly about its daily routine within our own bodies. It is truly fabulous.

PART III

The Rh Factor, Its Physical and Social Effects

NATURE abounds in strange paradoxes. Animals, impelled by craving for food absent from their diet, will eat their newborn offspring. Mother love, that strongest of human emotions, can sometimes be so repressed by unhappy circumstances that an unwanted child is brutally done away with. But the strangest paradox of all, it seems to me, is to be found in that grim phenomenon of a prospective mother being compelled, by a curious law of nature and against her most ardent wish, to destroy the infant she is carrying within her own body.

This is the cause of a disease of newborn infants known as erythroblastosis fetalis—sometimes called, more simply, hemolytic anemia of the newborn, or congenital hemolytic disease. The disease is fatal more often than not; and unfortunately it is confined to the offspring of certain mothers, frequently killing all their children except the first-born. This makes it a disease of some social importance, and it has been a real tragedy in many families.

This disease attacks the infant while it is yet in the mother's womb. Depending upon its severity, the pregnancy may end with a miscarriage, the infant may be born dead, or may succumb within a few days after birth. If the

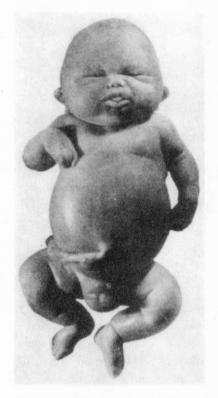

FIG. 11. FETUS WITH HYDROPIC (DROPSICAL) FORM OF ERYTHROBLASTOSIS FETALIS.

From *Rh*, by Edith L. Potter, 1947; with permission of the Year Book Publishers, Inc.

disease is exceptionally mild, the infant may survive after a period of illness.

One peculiarity of this disease is that the first-born infant is usually spared, but that either half or all of the subsequent children of the mother are often affected. All of the important facts about this disease—except its cause and prevention—have been known for some years.

In 1937, Landsteiner and Wiener, working upon an entirely different research problem, found that, when rabbits were injected with the red blood cells of rhesus monkeys, they produced antibodies in their blood which not only agglutinated the red cells of the monkey but also would agglutinate the red blood cells of about 85 percent of white people. They named this antigenic substance in the red cells of the monkey the Rh factor—using the first two letters of the zoological name of the species of monkey with which they were working. In 1939, Levine and Stetsen first related the Rh factor with stillbirth in infants; and, in 1941, showed that it was the cause of erythroblastosis.

The red blood cells of about 85 percent of white people contain the Rh factor; and it is absent from the blood of the remaining 15 percent. When present in the blood of an individual, he or she is said to be Rh-positive; and, when absent, Rh-negative. The pure Negro race is believed to be 100 percent Rh-positive; and, if a colored person be found to be Rh-negative, there is a strong presumption of admixture of white blood at some time in his ancestry.

The one essential condition that must be fulfilled in the production of erythroblastosis is that the fetus be Rh-positive and the mother Rh-negative. The reason for this will become apparent when we discuss the mechanism of the disease. If the mother be Rh-positive, the disease will not occur in the fetus, regardless of whether its blood is Rh-positive or Rh-negative.

Whether the fetus be Rh-positive or Rh-negative, when conceived in the uterus of an Rh-negative mother, depends upon the heredity of the father. If both parents of the father be Rh-negative, the father will be Rh-negative and the fetus, created by his union with the Rh-negative mother, will also be Rh-negative. The disease cannot occur under such circumstances.

If, however, the father is Rh-positive, he may be either homozygous or heterozygous with respect to his Rh-positiveness. Homozygous means that both his parents were Rh-positive, and that his inheritance of the Rh factor was from both of his parents. If he is heterozygous, it means that one of his parents was Rh-positive and the other Rh-negative—it matters not which was which—and he has inherited his Rh-positiveness from only one of his parents.

If the Rh-positive father be homozygous in this respect, all of the children of his union with an Rh-negative mother will be Rh-positive. In this case, the danger of the disease threatens most, if not all, the children of the union. If, however, he is heterozygous as regards the Rh factor, half of the children of such a union will be Rh-positive and half Rh-negative. In such a case, not more than half the children of the union—only the Rh-positive ones—will be in danger of the disease. Thus, the inheritance of the Rh factor follows Mendel's law.

Before discussing the mechanism of the production of erythroblastosis and of its prevention, it is necessary to digress for a moment to review briefly one of the immunologic reactions of the blood. In so doing, however, we shall undoubtedly, in the interest of simplicity, omit or distort certain facts that are not particularly germane to our purpose; and it is to be hoped that, realizing this, any immunologists who may read this discussion will temper their criticism accordingly.

For our purpose it is necessary to consider only one type of such defense reaction—the antigen-antibody reaction. An antigen is a foreign substance which, when introduced into a live animal, provokes a defense on the part of the body of the animal which takes the form of antibodies. Such antibodies are usually specific for the antigen which prompted their formation, and they render the antigen innocuous either by destroying it or by combining with it to form a harmless neutral substance. Certain tissues of the body have the power to produce antibodies when exposed to antigens; but this reaction is both more readily detectable and more accurately measurable in the blood than in other elements of the body.

Most antigens are either wholly protein or have a protein component. When of mixed composition, it is the protein fraction ordinarily that is antigenic and the other fraction that is toxic. In such cases, when it is possible to separate the toxic fraction from the protein fraction, the injection of the toxic fraction alone merely poisons the animal without stimulating the formation of antibodies against it; whereas the injection of the protein fraction will stimulate the production of antibodies, and will do so without poisoning the animal. The discovery of this principle has made possible the immunization of people against diphtheria and tetanus without danger—the complete toxins of each being highly poisonous.

The first injection of an antigen sets the reaction of antibody formation in motion. Nature believes in excessively adequate defenses, and always many more antibodies are produced than are necessary to combine the antigen that is injected. Successive injections of the antigen force even greater antibody production, until the animal often becomes immune even to huge doses of the toxic principle of the antigen. Antitoxins and other therapeutic sera are produced by the commercial application of this natural law. Animals, usually horses, are injected at intervals with increasing doses of toxic substances until their bloods abound in antibodies, at which time they are bled and their blood processed into therapeutic sera. In manufacturing diphtheria antitoxin, for example, diphtheria bacilli are grown in artificial media in which they produce large amounts of diphtheria toxin. This toxin is purified and used to inject horses. Since diphtheria toxin is highly poisonous, the initial doses are very small.

As the horse recovers from each dose of diphtheria toxin, it is given a larger dose. This is repeated until the horse has developed a high degree of immunity to diphtheria toxin. At this time, the horse is bled and the blood withdrawn is processed into diphtheria antitoxin which is injected into patients suffering from diphtheria. The horse's serum is heavily loaded with antibodies against diphtheria toxin, which neutralize the toxin in the patient's body by combining with it.

From this high point of antibody protection, which is reached shortly after the administration of the last dose of antigen, the antibodies slowly disappear from the blood if no further antigen is administered; and they may eventually disappear entirely so far as can be demonstrated. However, if, after their disappearance, another dose of the same antigen is administered, the antibodies reappear much more quickly than they appeared initially, and usually in greater numbers. This indicates that, once a body is sensitized to a particular antigen, it is, at least for a long time, on guard against that antigen, and keeps its war plan up to date for a speedy mobilization of its antibody force, even though it may maintain only a small standing army of antibodies during periods in which there is no threat.

As regards the causation of erythroblastosis, the Rh factor, carried in the red cells of the fetus, is the foreign substance, or antigen, which prompts the creation of the antibodies in the blood of the mother. It has heretofore been considered abnormal for a particle as large as a red blood cell to pass through the placenta from fetal to maternal circulation; but it is now obvious that something of this sort does occur in many cases—otherwise the mother's blood whould show no reaction to the Rh factor. It is essential to the disease that the Rh antigen in the red blood cells of the fetus get into the blood stream of the mother. If the fetal red cell does not itself cross the placental barrier, then the Rh antigen must be liberated into the blood serum of the fetus through the death of the red cells, and pass from the fetal to the maternal circulation in the same way that waste substances pass. As the mother builds up antibodies which combat the Rh factor, these in turn pass through the placenta into the blood of the fetus and destroy its red blood cells, thus producing the anemia in the fetus.

Apparently, in the usual case the amount of Rh antigen from the fetus that finds its way into the maternal bloodstream is small, for the production of antibodies is so slow and so limited that the first Rh-positive child of an Rh-negative mother ordinarily escapes the disease, or is affected so slightly that it survives without difficulty. However, the mother is sensitized during this first pregnancy; and, in subsequent pregnancies the anti-Rh antibodies are produced much more rapidly and in greater numbers, so that the danger to the infant increases greatly after the first pregnancy. Sometimes the second and third infant will survive. And there are Rh-negative mothers who bear a number of healthy Rh-positive children. In such cases it is a question as to whether the red cells of the fetuses fail to traverse the placental barrier to sensitize the mother, or whether the mother is one of those relatively rare individuals who is unable to form antibodies after stimulation with antigen.

While this explanation of the phenomenon of the reaction of an Rh-negative mother to her Rh-positive fetus is about as simple and nontechnical as is possible, it might clarify the mechanism if we indulged for a moment in an allegory. This allegory is the way an acquaintance of mine pictured the phenomenon after it had been explained to him.

Let us imagine a remote village in a far country, nestled in a peaceful valley surrounded by almost, but not quite, impassable mountains. The inhabitants of this village for generations have been completely isolated from the rest of the world. Those who have crossed the mountains have never returned. The inhabitants are kindly, industrious people. Crime is unknown in the village, and there has never been any necessity for a law enforcement agency. This village is the blood of the Rh-negative woman who has just become pregnant for the first time, and whose recently conceived and unborn child is Rh-positive. Her blood has not yet been exposed to the Rh factor. All the elements of her blood, as represented by the villagers, are at peace. She has not created a defense against the Rh factor because there has never been any reason to do so.

One year, a band of heavily armed, warlike Amazons settled on the far slope of one of the protecting mountains. They wandered up in the highest passes, where they met some of the villagers and arranged a sort of a trade agreement with them, but at first they made no effort to cross the mountain and descend into the valley of the village. But before long the Amazons became bolder; and singly and in small groups they did trespass into the village.

In this allegory, the warlike Amazons are the red blood cells of the fetus, carrying the Rh-factor. The pass in the mountain barrier is the placenta, where exchange occurs of various substances between the blood of the fetus and the blood of the mother. So long as the red blood cells of the fetus remain on their side of the mountain barrier and engage only in normal exchange at this point, peace prevails. But the intrusion of the armed invaders into the village creates quite a commotion.

The villagers became terribly alarmed over these forays by the Amazons, and hastily called a town meeting to discuss ways and means of defense against them. Had the Amazons come unarmed (that is, bearing no Rh factor), the villagers would have paid them scant attention; but the lethal weapons they bore terrified the villagers, and it was decided to organize a police force at once. When the size of the proposed police force was discussed, the wise counsel prevailed that it was better to have it too large than too small.

Being inexperienced in such matters, the villagers encountered some difficulty in getting their police force organized. The police, of course, are the antibodies against the Rh factor. These antibodies are first formed slowly and in small amount. Except for the purpose of allaying public excitement there was no urgent reason for haste, because the little invasions of the Amazons did small damage.

Just at the time when most of the obstacles to recruitment of the police force had been overcome and its ranks were swelling steadily, the Amazons suddenly moved away; and the threat to the peace of the village was ended. This symbolizes the termination of the first pregnancy. The villagers then slowly disbanded their police force; but filed away in the archives the perfected plan for the rapid mobilization of such a force against the day it would again be needed. With these allegorical pictures I have illustrated the steady increase in antibodies, and the fact that the red blood cells of the fetus are removed from contact, through birth of the child, before the antibodies are sufficient in quantity to cross the placental barrier and destroy the red cells of the child. Those red cells of the child, which get into the maternal circulation, are of course destroyed there; but this does no damage to either mother or child.

After the birth of the child—or the departure of the Amazon band—the antibodies, or police force, are greatly decreased; but one policeman is kept on duty against the return of the Amazons and around him another large force can be raised. This represents the reduced antibody titre in the mother's blood, and her sensitization to the Rh factor.

Sure enough, in a year or two the Amazons returned and took up their abode in the same old location just across the mountain. They resumed trade with the villagers at the summits of the passes, bartering odds and ends principally for food and building materials produced in the valley. This, of course, is a subsequent pregnancy in which the fetus is again Rh-positive while the mother must continue to be Rh-negative.

Again the Amazons began to sneak over the mountain and down into the village. But the villagers had profited by their first experience; and hasty reorganization of the police force was begun at once. Recruitment was rapid; and, for every policeman lost in encounters with the Amazons, there were three, or four, or five replacements. The police force grew in strength so rapidly that, in no time at all, scarcely had an Amazon crossed the mountain than she was set upon by the police and destroyed.

Still the recruitment of police went on; and soon the police were so strong that they were able not only to protect the village but, at the same time, to send detachments across the mountain to battle with the Amazons in their own territory. Many police were lost in these encounters, but the ranks were more than refilled by the recruiting program; and the battle in the territory of the Amazons continued until at last they went away again. Only a small number of Amazons escaped this time, and most of these were crippled from wounds received at the hands of the police. The mother's blood, having been sensitized by the first pregnancy, reacts much more rapidly, and builds up anti-Rh antibodies speedily and in quantity. Note that the Rh substances, in the form of Amazons, are this time almost immediately outnumbered by the mother's antibodies, in the form of police. Very shortly, the antibodies are so numerous that they can cross the placental barrier in quantity, and destroy the red cells of the fetus in the fetal circulation.

This, then is the mechanism of the production of the disease known as erythroblastosis, the pathology of which arises out of large-scale destruction of the red blood cells of the fetus by specific antibodies engendered in the circulation of the mother.

Until an effective means of preventing this serious disease has been discovered, this matter of the Rh factor presents a serious problem in marriage. An Rh-positive woman has nothing to worry about in this connection; but an Rh-negative woman, marrying an Rh-positive man, has to face the possibility of a large proportion of her pregnancies, after the first one at least, resulting in miscarriages or stillbirths, or in children who die in the first few weeks of life. The best she can hope for with an Rh-positive husband is that he is a heterozygote in this respect, which offers a fair chance of half of her pregnancies resulting in children with a good chance of survival.

There is some hope that a way of preventing such tragedies will be discovered before testing the blood of prospective brides and grooms for the Rh factor becomes a necessary procedure. If this hope does not materialize, a considerable number of otherwise desirable marriages either might have to be called off at no small emotional cost, or to be entered into with a poor prospect of rearing a healthy family.

A very great amount of research is being done in the effort to find a method of preventing the evil effects of the Rh factor other than by control of the mating of Rh-negative persons. Unfortunately, none has yet been reported which has been generally accepted by scientists and by practicing physicans.

At present, established treatment is limited to the replacement of the destroyed and damaged red cells of the newborn infant by transfusion with fresh blood. If the disease is not too severe, such transfusions will save the child.*

Once such a child recovers from erythroblastosis, it has nothing more to fear, itself, from the Rh factor during its life. As soon as it is old enough, however, if it be a male it should be informed that it is a heterozygous Rh-positive, and should, if possible, avoid mating with an Rh-negative female. So, having survived infancy, the Rh-positive child has no further concern for its own health because of its inheritance.

However, the Rh-negative child faces grave danger throughout life if he or she must ever receive a blood transfusion. Since blood transfusions are becoming increasingly frequent in the treatment of disease and injury, the possibility of encountering this danger at some time is not too remote. When an Rh-negative person receives a transfusion of Rh-positive blood, the same reaction occurs in the blood as occurs in that of an Rh-negative mother who is carrying an Rh-positive fetus—except that, since the amount of Rh antigen given in a blood transfusion is so many times greater than that carried in the fetal red cells that slip through the placental barrier, the formation of anti-Rh antibodies following transfusion is on an infinitely greater scale than it is during pregnancy.

As would be expected, the first transfusion of Rh-positive blood into an unsensitized Rh-negative person produces no visible reaction from this cause. If there is a reaction, it

* A most important scientific observation was announced after this volume was set in type. This is to the effect that, for transfusion of newborn infants suffering from erythroblastosis fetalis, the blood of female donors is much more effective than that of male donors. This suggests the presence of some protective substance against Rh antibodies in the blood of women which is absent from, or in lesser concentration in, the blood of men.

is due to a cause or causes other than the Rh factor. However, anti-Rh antibodies are produced in great quantities following this first transfusion, and a second transfusion of Rh-positive blood some days later ordinarily will produce a very severe and often fatal reaction from the agglutination of the Rh-positive red cells of the donor by the antibodies in the serum of the Rh-negative recipient.

Herein also lies great danger for the Rh-negative mother, immediately or recently delivered of an Rh-positive infant. If she has been heavily sensitized during her pregnancy—regardless of whether or not her infant was affected—a transfusion of Rh-positive blood may result fatally. The antibodies in her own blood will destroy the red cells in the transfused blood, causing a reaction that may result in her death. Since transfusion of the mother is occasionally indicated after delivery, this is a danger that must be guarded against.

Thousands upon thousands of blood transfusions were given to American soldiers in the European Theater of Operations during the late war. Only O-type blood—from so-called universal donors—was used. But, since the Rh factor was a relatively new discovery requiring further study, since the testing of donors for this factor was, at that time, a practical impossibility, and since soldiers had not been tested in Europe because of the very small amount of testing serum available in the world, the Rh factor was disregarded in transfusion.

It was commonly noted in that theater of war that severe reactions rarely followed the first transfusion, or even the fourth or fifth transfusion if they were all given within a very short period. However, subsequent transfusions after intervals of five to ten days were much more prone to produce severe reactions than initial transfusions. This phenomenon gave us confidence in the purity of the blood we were using, since defective blood would have produced reactions whenever it was used—first or later.

Many soldiers died shortly after transfusions, but almost all of them died of their injuries and not as the result of the transfusion. In less than ten cases, however, out of the thousands of transfusions, we decided, after careful autopsy, that the cause of death was the reaction following blood transfusion. In all of these cases there had been previous transfusions some days before. The findings at autopsy were typical of destruction of red blood cells upon a large scale. In the light of research done since that time, the Rh factor seems to be the most probable cause of these fatal reactions. Each death of this kind is a tragedy which profoundly moves the medical man who was unable to prevent it. From the broad point of view, however, these few accidental deaths were, perhaps, not too great a price to pay for the thousands of other lives saved only by transfusions of this blood.

There are no insurmountable obstacles to guarding against this danger in civil life. Donors can be tested, as well as typed, for the Rh factor. It will require that blood banks stock twice as many kinds of blood as formerly, unless only O-type Rh-negative blood is used. If exact matching is followed, there will have to be A-type blood Rh-positive, and A-type blood Rh-negative, and so on through the four types of blood. In any event, no Rh-negative person must ever be given a transfusion with Rh-positive blood—with the possible exception of the first transfusion in his life and then only in an urgent emergency.

In the case of an Rh-negative mother, even the first transfusion of Rh-positive blood is very dangerous.

However, the Rh factor has introduced a serious element in the wholesale use of whole blood in war casualties. The stockage and distribution of a single type of blood is a difficult matter; and, if both Rh-positive and Rh-negative blood are required, the problem will be quite complicated. We must hope that research will soon offer a solution for this complex problem.

A number of other antigen-antibody reactions in blood have been described, and more are being discovered each day. None other, thus far, has produced such profound effects as have those arising out of blood types and the Rh factor. As the science of biochemistry advances it may become possible to synthetize inhibiting substances to prevent these dangerous reactions. Until that time the only protection lies in avoiding the mixing of incompatible bloods. One of the great biological manufacturers is now attempting to synthetize such a substance. If and when this is accomplished, this treatment will be plentiful and cheap.

MODERN SURGERY OF THE HEART AND LUNGS

Surgery of the heart and great vessels. "Blue baby" operations. Lung surgery in cancer and tuberculosis. Motion pictures of actual surgery of the heart

THORACIC SURGERY, or the surgery of the chest, is the youngest yet most precocious of the special fields of surgical endeavor.

The great milestones in the evolution of surgery are too numerous and too complex to outline fully, but certainly we cannot omit anesthesia. The horrors of surgery without pain control are suggested by the fact that, until the middle of the last century, operating theaters had to be placed at a point far removed from the hospital beds. Pain control was, at best, poor and incomplete when limited to the effects produced by hashish, opiates, and whisky. Control of pain began with general anesthesia or with those anesthetics that put the patient to sleep. More specific control is acquired when a part of the patient is made insensible by local or spinal injection of anesthetics.

The control of infection and of pain introduced new eras of surgery. It became possible to operate within the abdomen or head, but the chest remained invulnerable until very recently.

The barriers to successful surgery in the chest stemmed from inability to maintain the essential respiratory action of the lungs when the chest wall was opened, since the lungs are not attached to the chest wall but are suspended freely within this closed cavity, inflating and deflating as the pressure within the cavity varies from negative to positive with the expansion and contraction of the chest cavity. As soon as the chest was opened the lungs collapsed and they no longer maintained the oxygen life line. Surgeons tried to work in closed vacuum chambers that maintained the rhythmic expansion of the functioning lung, but this was unsatisfactory. Finally, the expedient of placing a tight tube in the patient's trachea or windpipe gave the needed control. This permitted of preventing the collapse of the lungs by positive pressure applied through their own air passages and made them independent of the normal partial vacuum within the chest cavity. Anesthetic agents and oxygen could be given in measured amounts. One man, the anesthesiologist, could now assume control of the other man's, the patient's, breathing while that patient was asleep with his chest open. Oxygen and other gases could be delivered at any desired rate. The door was open for surgery within the chest.

The opportunity for surgical intervention within the chest having been provided, a host of disorders presented themselves. Congenital abnormalities or disorders with which people were born, such as cysts, tumors, or hernias (for example, the upside-down stomach) in the chest could be removed or repaired.

Lung tissue could now be removed. Infections and cancer are the principal offenders that indicate excision of lung tissue itself. The offending infections are of many kinds. At times, the finer air passages become dilated, functionless, and the seat of foul infections. This disease is called bronchiectasis. Sometimes abscesses in the lung can behave in a similar fashion. The tragic physical and social implications of a person overburdened by infection and racked by cough productive of foul sputum need only be suggested to be appreciated. Such conditions may be responsible for chronic or even fatal illness, divorce, or suicide. The precise anatomical removal of such diseased tissues by the thoracic surgeon spells the emancipation and rehabilitation of these unfortunate patients.

Certain forms of tuberculosis lend themselves to lobectomy (the removal of a lobe) or even pneumonectomy (the removal of an entire lung).

Up to the present time, the only satisfactory treatment for cancer is total excision. The ability to operate within the chest extends such surgery to the lung where a lung or a portion of lung containing cancer can be removed. Cancers of the lung are far from uncommon; and the outlook for such patients was hopeless until extensive thoracic surgery became possible. Also such surgery of removal can be applied to the esophagus, the tube carrying food from the mouth to the stomach. This remarkable surgery of the esophagus can be performed without interference with the patient's ability to eat normally following the operation. A tube is made of the stomach to replace that part of the esophagus removed because of the cancer.

In some ways, surgery of the heart is the most difficult, if not the most delicate, of all surgery. The greatest source of difficulty is that it is impossible to suspend the active operation of the heart during the time it is being worked upon. One does not do surgery of the stomach while it is digesting a meal, nor amputate a leg during a footrace; nor does one expect a motor mechanic to grind a valve or tighten a bearing while the motor is running at high speed. Yet this is exactly what the thoracic surgeon is called upon to do in surgery of the heart and great vessels adjacent to the heart; and he has developed remarkable ingenuity in doing extraordinary things to the heart without, so to speak, letting it miss a single beat.

Surgery of the heart and great vessels would be relatively simple if the circulation of the blood could be suspended for a reasonable period. Except for one organ, circulation could be suspended for as long as 30 minutes without fatal effect upon the patient. The exception is the brain; and the brain cannot survive longer than eight minutes without a constant supply of blood. Irreparable brain damage has resulted from depriving the brain of its oxygen supply for even shorter periods. For this reason, any surgery which requires interference with the blood supply of the brain must be done most expeditiously.

The greater part of the surgery of the great vessels near the heart is done to correct congenital defects and anomalies. In addition to the accidents of growth in the fetus, which may occur in any part of any organ of the body, there is one accident of adjustment from intra-uterine life to free living in the world that is peculiar to the great vessels near the heart.

At this point it may help if we pause to review the high points of the circulation of the blood in the free-living human body. The circulation of the blood is divided between two separate and distinct circulatory systems—the pulmonary and the systemic. The systemic veins collect the exhausted blood from all parts of the body except the lungs, and empty it into the right side of the heart. The right ventricle then pumps it into the lungs through the pulmonary artery. In the lungs, this depleted blood is aerated, in which process it gives up its waste products and takes on a fresh supply of oxygen.

Now ready again to supply the body tissues, the renovated blood returns to the left side of the heart through the pulmonary vein. The left ventricle then pumps it into the systemic arteries through the aorta.

It is apparent that, with such a mechanism, there must be a perfect balance between the pulmonary and systemic circulations. This is to say that the right side of the heart cannot pump more blood into the lungs than can be disposed of by the left side of the heart after aeration. On the other hand, the left side of the heart can supply no more blood to the rest of the body than is returned to it from the pulmonary circulation. So, in the free-living body, the amount of blood sent to the lungs by the right side of the heart at every heart-beat is, within insignificant compensating differences, exactly the same as is pumped out to the body by the left side of the heart at the same heart-beat. Otherwise, after a few beats of the heart, the blood would all be either in the systemic or the pulmonary circulation, depending upon which side of the heart was operating at the greater capacity.

The infant does not engage in respiration until after birth. During the entire period of development within the uterus, it receives its oxygen supply, as well as its food supply, and disposes of its waste products, through the maternal circulation by means of a mechanism of exchange of these substances through the placenta. For this reason, the lungs of the fetus are compressed and wholly inactive insofar as respiration is concerned. The only necessity for blood in the lungs of the fetus is for their own nourishment since no oxygen-carbon dioxide exchange takes place in the lungs until after the newborn infant begins to breathe.

Since the amount of blood pumped by the right side of the heart into the lungs of the fetus before birth is limited not only by the necessity for blood in the lungs but more especially by the amount that the compressed lungs can accommodate, and since the amount of blood pumped to the growing fetal body is limited to that returned from the lungs to the left side of the heart, one of two situations must obtain. Either the amount of blood furnished the rest of the body must be limited to the small amount passing through the compressed lungs, or there must be a by-pass through which some of the blood leaving the right ventricle can reach the systemic circulation without passing through the lungs of the fetus.

Nature has provided just such a by-pass. In the fetus there is a blood vessel which connects the pulmonary artery with the aorta. Known as the ductus arteriosus, it operates in this way: the right ventricle at each beat pumps considerably more blood than the fetal lungs can accommodate. The blood vessels in the lungs are filled, and the excess, before reaching the lungs, flows through the ductus arteriosus and joins the outgoing blood leaving the left side of the heart en route to all parts of the body except the lungs. This arrangement permits an adequate supply of blood to the growing body of the fetus, and, more important, it permits the development of the right side of the fetal heart to the size that will be necessary when large amounts of blood must pass through the lungs as respiration is established. Thus, in the fetus, the right ventricle assists the left ventricle in supplying the systemic circulation, and both sides of the heart grow and develop rather evenly.

One of the first questions which may occur to you is, what happens after the birth—does not this by-pass continue to reduce the amount of blood passing through the lungs? In the normal infant it does not, and the reason is some of the most clever engineering in all nature.

As we have explained, the chest cavity of the fetus is much smaller than that of the infant because there is no respiration. The diaphragm rests higher in the fetus, and the heart of the fetus lies higher than it will lie after respiration is established. So, with the first breath that the newborn infant takes, not only is the chest wall expanded but also the diaphragm is pulled sharply downward. This descent of the diaphragm, together with the expansion of the lungs through inflation, forces the heart and the great vessels downward. Curiously enough, the heart does not descend in its original plane, but rotates somewhat in its descent.

This rotation of the heart and the great vessels near it twists the ductus arteriosus and closes it, just as you can close a soft rubber tube by twisting it. After it is closed and no longer functioning, the ductus arteriosus goes the way of all living flesh that is no longer useful. It degenerates and persists in the body only as a small strip of connective tissue with the lumen completely obliterated.

The process we have just considered is the normal process. Occasionally something goes wrong with this delicate mechanism, and the ductus arteriosus fails to close when the heart descends. This leaves open the direct passage between the aorta and the pulmonary artery. Whereas in the fetus, with the limited capacity of the lungs, the flow in the ductus arteriosus is from the pulmonary artery to the aorta, now that the pulmonary circulation has been opened up by respiration, the higher pressure in the aorta forces some of the systemic blood back into the pulmonary artery and lungs.

In such a situation, the left side of the heart is forced to pump from two to four times the amount of blood required in the systemic circulation, depending upon the amount of the leakage through the ductus arteriosus. The volume of leak may vary between 45 percent and 75 percent of the total amount of blood discharged from the left ventricle.

This excess work required of the left ventricle forces it to enlarge. It may cause failure of the heart and death. It ordinarily restricts to a greater or lesser degree the amount of exertion the child or adult can tolerate, since exertion increases the demand for blood in the systemic circulation. However, many mild cases live a long and useful life without too serious restriction of activity; and a few are even able to indulge in athletic sports. It all depends upon the volume of the leak.

When this condition is of a severity that threatens life or restricts activity to an intolerable degree, the chest can be opened and the ductus arteriosus closed with sutures. Simple ligation, or tying it off, is considered by some surgeons not to be satisfactory for the reason that too often it reopens after a time; however, the operation of choice must be selected in each case after the anatomical situation has been determined at first hand.

The other common malformations of the great vessels around the heart are coarctation of the aorta and pulmonary stenosis. Recent advances in surgery have brought a considerable degree of relief to both these conditions, which have hitherto been unapproachable.

Coarctation of the aorta is a localized constriction of the

aorta at, or just below, the junction of the ductus arteriosus. As you might expect, this increases the resistance of the aorta, and forces extra work upon the left side of the heart in the raising of the pressure necessary to get a sufficient volume of blood through the constriction. At present, the operation of preference for this condition is one of cutting out the constricted portion and joining the severed ends of the aorta together. This sounds simple, but, when you realize that this means cutting the main outlet of the heart while the heart continues to beat, and doing a watertight job of stitching this great artery together again—all without a fatal loss of blood and within the preciously little time that circulation to the brain can be suspended—the tremendous skill required becomes apparent.

Of all the surgery of the heart and great vessels, operations for the relief of pulmonary stenosis have had the most publicity. Pulmonary stenosis is a narrowing of the opening between the pulmonary artery and the right ventricle of the heart. The so-called "blue babies," to which the lay press has devoted much space of late, are sufferers from pulmonary stenosis.

The effect of the constriction of the entrance into the pulmonary artery is, in general, like that of the constriction of any blood vessel—of coarctation of the aorta, for example. It limits the volume of blood which can pass in a given time at a given pressure. It forces the creation of higher pressures to get a required volume of blood through; and this throws just that more work upon the heart with resultant hypertrophy and danger of failure. One difference between pulmonary stenosis and coarctation of the aorta is that, in the former, it is principally the right side of the heart that is overworked, whereas in the latter the heavy burden falls on the left ventricle.

The correction of this condition by surgery lies in connecting a pulmonary artery with an adjacent systemic artery. This permits a part of the pulmonary circulation to be furnished from the systemic circulation, thus reducing the volume of blood which has to be forced through the constricted pulmonary artery. In effect, this operation creates a patent ductus arteriosus—the principal difference being that one of the larger branches of the aorta is used rather than the aorta itself. Obviously, such an operation does not cure the condition, but ameliorates it by shifting a part of the excessive burden of the right ventricle upon the left. At best, such patients become comparable to those with a patent ductus arteriosus in which the leak is small. In this operation, also, more than ordinary speed, skill, and dexterity are necessary for success.

I have mentioned the necessity for speed in all surgical procedures which require interruption of the circulation to the brain. This places a limit upon the extent of the surgery that can be attempted upon the heart and great vessels around the heart.

If only some method can be devised to replace temporarily the heart and lungs, the limits of permissible surgery in the chest will be greatly extended. Several apparatuses have been devised to do this. The latest one is that of Dr. Clarence Crafoord, of Stockholm. This machine receives the venous blood returning toward the heart, aerates it, and pumps it into the aorta. In this way both the heart and lungs are by-passed—the machine fulfilling the functions of both. This apparatus is still in the experimental stage and has not, to my knowledge, been employed upon man.

I regret very much that it is impossible to reproduce in print the magnificent motion pictures shown at this lecture by Dr. Dwight E. Harken, of the faculty of Harvard Medical School and of the staff of the Peter Bent Brigham Hospital, in Boston.

Doctor Harken served as Chief of one of the Thoracic Surgery Centers in the European Theater of Operations during World War II. One of the films, which he showed during this lecture, was that of an operation for the removal of a piece of shell fragment from the left ventricle of a wounded soldier. The other film showed the correction of a congenital defect (patent ductus arteriosus) in a pregnant woman who had hitherto been able to enjoy fair health despite the handicap, but whose heart was unable to perform the added work required in nourishing her unborn child. The operation was successful and the pregnancy continued without interruption.

The photography (in color) is first-class, and the audience was able to see every detail of the operations. Doctor Harken's contribution was a rare treat, which those in attendance fully appreciated.

It is because of especially skilled medical men like Doctor Harken—and there are many—that so few American wounded died of their wounds in the late war, and that the American people enjoy the finest medical care in the world. Such skills can be produced in quantity only in a free medical profession; they have always disappeared from medicine controlled by government. I am confident that those who witnessed this demonstration of medical care of superior quality (and I wish that more of my fellow citizens could have such an opportunity) want no regimentation of medicine in this country.

MODERN PREVENTION AND TREATMENT OF MENTAL DISEASE

From Bedlam to thalamotomy. Psychotherapy, shock therapy and psychosurgery, including prefrontal lobotomy, topectomy and thalamotomy

In RESPONSE TO MacBeth's inquiry about Lady MacBeth's health, the doctor replied that she was

> Not so sick, my lord,
> As she is troubled with thick-coming fancies
> That keep her from her rest.

With a layman's confidence in medical skill, MacBeth orders the doctor to

> Cure her of that.
> Cans't thou not minister to a mind diseas'd,
> Pluck from the memory a rooted sorrow,
> Raze out the written troubles of the brain,
> And with some sweet oblivious antidote
> Cleanse the stuff'd bosom of that perilous stuff
> Which weighs upon the heart?

Had this setting been of today, the doctor, if he were a psychiatrist, would have held out hope. But this eleventh century physician was forced to reply sadly,

> Therein the patient   –
> Must minister to himself.

This confession of medical impotence in the field of mental illness expresses the helplessness of psychiatry until recent times. Nothing was known of the causes of mental illness and little more of the treatment. In fact, almost all the treatment practiced was mistreatment.

Mistreatment of mental illness seems to be a product of civilization. Among most primitive peoples, the psychotic person enjoyed unusual privileges. He was regarded as a special ward of the Deity, and his harmless aberrations and even antisocial conduct were regarded with amused tolerance or sympathetic forbearance.

When developing civilization produced concepts of abstract good and evil—weighed in the arbitrary scales of theology—there was evolved the first classification of mental illness. The average man, in his inveterate egotism, regarded himself as mentally normal, whether or not he would admit to being mentally average. He was his own master, and was in full control of his person. Since the concept of a sick mind was beyond his comprehension, and since he believed fully in all kinds of spirits, it was natural that he attributed mental illness to the possession of the body by a foreign spirit—a definite entity, even though intangible, which had overcome the proper ego of the body and had taken over the direction of the actions of that body.

Depending upon the direction given the captivated body, the spirit was either a good or an evil one. Among the ancient Jews, evil spirits were devils; and those unfortunates who were unable, because of mental illness, to conduct themselves within the established code, were believed to be possessed by devils.

The tortures inflicted upon these afflicted persons, in well-intentioned efforts to drive out the devils, were in keeping with the cruelty of the age. Thus did psychotherapy begin. There is one thing to be said for these misguided efforts—the treatment, however brutal, was of short duration; and the total of the mistreatment was far less than that practiced centuries later in the mere confinement of such wretches for the remainder of their lives.

As the social organization became more complex and more demanding, all mentally ill, whether possessed by good or by evil spirits, became nuisances; and society, no longer tolerant of even harmless aberrations, developed institutions in which to incarcerate them. One of the most famous of these early lunatic asylums, as they were known even unto our own day, was Bethlehem Hospital, in London —which, with the curious gift of the English for corruption of pronunciation, soon became Bedlam. That "bedlam" was incorporated into our language to denote "a place or scene of uproar and confusion" is eloquent evidence of conditions within this so-called hospital.

So lacking in sensitiveness to human suffering were the Londoners of the fourteenth to the seventeenth centuries that the inmates of Bedlam were regarded as unwilling clowns, and the multitude paid admission to watch their antics.

While the conditions within mental hospitals were somewhat improved over the centuries, the institution continued to be regarded as the only suitable place for the care of the mentally ill. That country was backward which provided insufficient institutional facilities to care for all of its mentally ill. There are many such countries in the world—in fact, no country, not even our own, which is more generous than most, yet has sufficient institutional beds for the care of its psychotics. In the United States, it is customary to confine them in jails until an institutional bed becomes available. In Central America, I have seen them shackled and chained to the wall in private homes.

The evolution of psychiatry followed the general pattern of the development of all science. First, there was the establishment of criteria for the recognition of mental disease. At first crude, and generally restricted to obvious antisocial actions dangerous or annoying to others, these criteria have been partially refined, and are being constantly extended. Well within our lifetime there have been admitted to the field of mental illness many conditions which hitherto had been entirely overlooked or had been explained upon purely physical grounds.

Next came classification; and, in my student days, classification of mental illness was the limit of both diagnosis and treatment. There was no treatment worthy of the name—not even for the mental illness resulting from syphilis of the brain (general paralysis of the insane, or paresis) because there was no adequate treatment for syphilis. And, even after systemic syphilis could be treated with fair success, the disease could not be controlled once it affected the central nervous system. The medical students of my day, mostly imbued with a desire to relieve some of the suffering of humanity, often wondered why any physician selected psychiatry as a specialty, since there was so little that could be done for such patients.

Because psychiatry was, and still is to a lesser degree, an inexact science, classifications of mental illness changed almost as often, and almost as radically, as ladies' fashions. The classification that I learned as a medical student has been changed several times; but of much greater importance, it has been enlarged to include mental illnesses of less obvious character, perhaps, but of greater social importance.

New additions to the family of mental illnesses are the psychoneuroses, which were extensively publicized during the late war. The term "psychoneuroses" was for a time a catchall expression to classify almost all mental illnesses of a gravity less than that of the major psychoses.

I do not intend to enter into a detailed discussion of the personality, and the character and behavior disorders, which make up the great bulk of mental illness not treated in psychiatric institutions. In many ways these are the most important of all mental illnesses. While usually they are less incapacitating in the individual case than a major psychosis, in the aggregate they are responsible for a tremendous amount of suffering, of loss of efficiency, and of economic waste.

For example, one of these disorders is what is rapidly becoming known as psychosomatic illness. The proportion of people seeking medical aid for physical symptoms, who have no organic basis for their complaints, is not known. The head of a very large and reputable clinic recently told me that 50 percent of the patients coming to his clinic had no organic disease whatsoever; their troubles were entirely disorders of the mind. An additional 25 percent, said he, had organic troubles of such insignificant character and import that they would not have sought medical aid except for the complicating mental condition. These estimates have been agreed to by many experienced physicians. This fact is of the greatest importance in considering all proposals for national health insurance.

As Dr. Daniel Blain has pointed out, until quite recently our entire need in the field of treatment of mental illness has been measured in terms of hospital beds. A recent report of the Commissioner of Mental Hospitals of the State of New York included these words: "I call your attention to the increasing number of admissions to our hospitals. It is obvious that more hospital beds will have to be built and a long-range plan developed in this regard." He mentioned no other method of attack upon mental illness; and, perhaps in some part because of this method of attack, more than one-half of the hospital beds in the United States are now occupied by patients suffering from mental illness.

Because of the shortage of psychiatric beds, and of adequately trained personnel of all categories in the field of mental health, emphasis has recently been placed upon intensive treatment of the more serious psychoses as well as of the milder forms of mental illness. It is a curious fact that, so long as facilities for the housing of mental patients were reasonably adequate, we were content to solve the problem by incarcerating them in such institutions. The shortage of beds, as well as of competent personnel, stimulated intensive treatment in order that beds could be freed for new patients. The results of much of this intensive treatment have been impressive.

The shortage of psychiatric beds for veterans was particularly acute, and intensive treatment was pushed vigorously. The partial success, which was early evident, stimulated the medical service of the Veterans' Administration to greater efforts. It was through the simple, but slow and arduous, means of plugging every hole in every hospital, working here and there with limited staffs to accomplish better intensive treatment, that the unexpected and unhoped-for result was finally achieved of discharging more psychiatric patients in one month than were admitted in that period. Since that time, approximately a year ago, this goal has been achieved month after month, until now relatively few more beds are needed to take care of the service-connected load of veterans with mental disease than were needed when the veteran population was much smaller. Treatment results can be stated generally in terms of World War II veterans who have received intensive treatment in the early stages of mental illness; and, at the present time, approximately 75 percent of all new cases are discharged from the hospitals in good condition by the end of three months. Intensive treatment has benefited World War I and other veterans as well, as evidenced by the fact that out of fifty-five hundred neuropsychiatric patients discharged from hospitals in one of the late months of record, over seventeen hundred were veterans of World War I, in their fifties or older, all of whom had been in the hospital for some years.

The next stage in the progress toward preventive aspects was to treat the disease earlier; and here was found a characteristic development which began about the same time as the effort to intensify the treatment in hospitals— namely, the creation of ways and means of getting patients before they were forced to enter hospitals, largely through what are known as mental hygiene clinics. This movement had started many years ago with the birth of the mental hygiene movement, initiated by Clifford Beers, a cured patient from a mental hospital; but it had been slow in taking root throughout the country, impeded as it was by small interest and by a lack of vision on the part of those responsible for solving the problem of mental disease and personality disorder. How successful the mental hygiene

clinics of the Veterans' Administration have been thus far
is shown by the estimates of a number of qualified observers, that between 25 and 40 percent of the 14,500
veterans now seen per month in these clinics were patients
who would have had to be hospitalized had not this out-
patient treatment been available. The average number of
visits for the patients in the mental hygiene clinics has been
less than six, which means that for a relative cost of six
times $5.75—in other words, for slightly less than $35—men
have been saved from entering hospitals where, once having crossed this Rubicon, they might stay anywhere from
three months to thirty years, at a cost of $5.00 to $10 per
day, depending upon the hospital. This is a small part of
the total price the country has been paying, when it is
considered that whole families frequently are disorganized,
and sometimes wholly dissolved by the mental illness of
one member, and that the communities are losing the benefit of workers both in the family and in productive plants.

Among these developments in the gradual extension of
real treatment in psychiatry from the hospitalized psychotic
to the more mildly ill individual who is treated outside of
hospitals, there has come a deepening realization of the
importance of psychologic difficulties arising from situations
which, though not strictly medical, have been closely allied
to the medical field. Largely in the field of human relations,
mental illness often numbers its victims among the so-called
normal members of society. The Federal Security Agency
has estimated that there are approximately eight million
persons in the United States who either have suffered or
are suffering from mental disease or personality disorder.
This amounts to over 5 percent of the total population.
Obviously, most of these are not listed as patients in either

hospital or mental hygiene clinic. They are carrying on their work or other activities with these handicaps in the best way they know, sometimes carrying a recognized burden in the face of handicaps known and understood by their acquaintances. At other times, much more complex disorders have caused people to become difficult, irresponsible, or childish—a drag upon their communities rather than sharers in the problems common to all. Psychiatry is now recognized to be related to the problems which cause delinquency and to all stages of criminology, where the constitutional psychopath finds his greatest field for self-expression. Psychiatric conditions are related to the breakdown of family life, where maladjustment plays a major part in the increasing divorce rate. The psychologic elements in teaching, among both students and teachers, have, in many instances, caused serious failure in teaching systems. Failure of some sort related to this field is clearly connected with the present decline in the influence of the church. The great subject of leadership—and its first cousin, morale—is composed, in part, of psychologic ingredients, frequently tinged with the presence or absence of psychiatric difficulties. World War II, with its strenuous efforts toward scientific principles of selection, demonstrated the number of defects of this nature in people who were considered average citizens and who had been carrying on without recognition of the difficulties under where they were laboring. The number of men rejected for psychologic causes is still one of the great disappointments in this survey of manpower for the armed forces.

In discussing the purely preventive phases of psychiatry, it must be admitted that even those most interested in the subject have not yet arrived at methods comparable to the immunization methods which have proved so successful in many somatic diseases. While much is known concerning the influences which combine to cause and promote mental and personality disorders, much preventive work still remains to be done in the fields of persuasion, education, and the forces which produce maturity of the personality.

As knowledge has expanded in the field of mental disease, so has treatment been enlarged. One of the most used methods of treatment, and one of relatively recent development, is psychotherapy. A strict definition of "psychotherapy" is treatment by psychology; but, in its application, the term has been broadened to include all methods and devices used to improve the psychological aspects of the patient's illness, including both the simpler procedures of suggestion, instruction, counsel and advice, as well as the complex techniques of psychoanalysis and hypnosis.

Much of the value of psychotherapy depends upon the patient's own contributions to the treatment. Great benefit is experienced from the patient's own disclosure of his emotional conflicts and his delusions. Psychotherapy can be given individually or in small groups. Group psychotherapy is economical of the time of trained personnel; and, in certain conditions, has proved more productive than individual treatment. Once the inhibitions of the group can be broken down, and their fears and anxieties exposed, the individual patients derive great assistance from the realization that others are suffering in a like manner. Often the group keeps the discussion active, and the psychiatrist does not have to make much of a contribution. Thousands of people in the United States are attending such sessions regularly, and are thereby able to continue productive occupations.

In very recent years, psychoanalysis has grown in favor among better psychiatrists. Like many other worthy techniques, its reputation has suffered through exploitation by incompetent and unscrupulous charlatans. In certain circles, made up of people with more money than brains, to be psychoanalyzed has become a mark of social distinction. Fashionable poseurs, some of whom have never had any medical training whatsoever, are plucking these shallow-brained geese for all the traffic will bear. In this racket, a foreign name and a foreign origin seem to be tangible assets of great value. There are many Americans who like to believe that Europe is still the fountain of all medical knowledge. They are unaware that the world capital of medicine moved westward across the Atlantic more than twenty-five years ago; and that it is likely to remain in this country unless we, too, drive it out through foolish experimentation in the field of medical economics. That is largely what drove it out of Europe. If we ape Europe in this—as we seem to be doing in other fields of politics—we shall lose our present preeminent position in medicine.

Psychoanalysis grew out of the work of Freud. He used the term initially to denote a method of treatment of mental illness. As Dr. William C. Menninger points out, much of the criticism of Freud is the result of a want of understanding of his work, even among psychiatrists; and that many psychiatrists, who openly disagree with Freud's observations and conclusions, utilize his techniques in the diagnosis and treatment of mental illness.

"One of the most significant discoveries of psychoanalysis was that the events of infancy and babyhood are all-important in shaping the personality or character of the individual. Psychoanalysis turned the spotlight, perhaps, better, the telescope, on this area of development and has shown without question or doubt that it is during these early years that the basic personality structure and patterns of behavior are laid down. It is during this period that the groundwork is laid for later mental health or ill health. Since this experience occurs during a period for which the adult has amnesia [i.e., a loss of memory by the conscious mind, however the forgotten events may be indelibly impressed upon the subconscious mind], he is completely unable to explain certain attitudes or behavior in himself. . . .

"One of the most frequent criticisms of psychoanalysis is that it is too much occupied with sex. Critics are unaware, however, of the fact that to Freud the term 'sex' meant far more than genital activity. It included all forms of physical gratification. Moreover, few of these critics know that every psychiatric patient under intensive psychological treatment always brings up this subject himself. The treatment of patients led to the discovery that seeking for gratification is an instinctive drive in every person and cannot be ignored because of prudishness any more than can any other instinctive need. . . . Sexual maladjustment is accepted, even by nonpsychoanalytic psychiatrists, as a major causative factor in mental illness. . . . Incidentally, the American cultural taboo against discussion of this instinctual need is a significant factor in the high incidence of neuroses. . . .

"The second major contribution of psychoanalytic psychiatry to the understanding of behavior is a concept of the anatomy of the personality as being divided into a conscious and an unconscious portion. None of us have clear recollections of those experiences in infancy that occurred during psychosexual development. Thus none of us have any real knowledge of the basis of many of our most outstanding personality traits—honesty or dishonesty, sociability, selfishness or unselfishness, and so forth. The average individual usually believes that he knows why he does all that he does. Sometimes, however, his explanations for his attitudes and behavior are so shallow that he himself may question their validity. Occasionally he may admit that he does not know just why he does a certain thing or why he takes a certain point of view. Human behavior is complex, and the average person has no explanation why one individual has a persistent fear of crowded places or another has frank delusions. The same would puzzle the psychiatrist without a theory of the existence of a major part of the personality—the unconscious—that motivates much of our behavior." [1]

So much for what might be called the medical treatment of mental illness. It is a popular fantasy, frequently revived when some antisocial individual runs afoul the law, that abnormal conduct is the result of some pressure somewhere upon the brain which can be relieved by an operation. It is true that occasionally a brain tumor produces psychotic symptoms; but, other than being a frequent cause of epileptic seizures, such removable growths play no very important role in behavior for longer than a few months.

However, in very recent years, both physical medicine and surgery have been brought into the armamentarium of the psychiatrist. Some years ago, a German psychiatrist made the observation that epileptics never suffered from schizophrenia—or, conversely, that schizophrenics never had

[1] *Psychiatry,* by William C. Menninger, M.D., Cornell University Press, Ithaca, 1948. Reprinted by permission of the publishers. If any of my readers are interested in pursuing this subject further I recommend not only this work but also Dr. Menninger's *You and Psychiatry;* both books are written for nonmedical readers.

epileptic seizures. From this he reasoned that recurrent convulsive seizures might have an inhibiting effect upon the development of this type of psychosis.

This psychiatrist began experimenting with the artificial production of convulsive seizures in psychotic individuals. In the early work, a drug, metrazol, was used to induce convulsions. The effect of this drug was reasonably satisfactory except for one unfortunate side-reaction—just prior to loss of consciousness and the onset of the convulsions, the patient experienced a terrifying sensation of impending dissolution. He remembered this sensation after his return to consciousness; and the experience engendered, in many patients, an intense fear and dislike of the treatment. This reaction to the treatment was a handicap, and other methods of producing convulsions with reasonable safety were sought.

The next development in shock therapy was the use of insulin. It is well known that large doses of insulin, by lowering the sugar content of the blood, induce convulsions. Insulin is now used extensively, especially in cases in which it is desirable to limit the violence of the convulsions or to produce a mild state of shock with few or no convulsive seizures. This limited treatment is known as sub-insulin shock.

The third method to be used was the momentary passage through the brain, from side to side, of a very high voltage and very low amperage electric current. This is known as electroshock, and continues to be widely used; it is probably the method of preference. Electroshock has the advantage of leaving no unpleasant memories behind. Ordinarily, patients have no fear of the treatment and, even when severely psychotic, will cooperate in it.

Until recently, there was one particular danger in shock treatment. The convulsions often were so severe that the patient injured himself. The terrific pull of muscles undergoing such uncontrolled spasmodic seizures was occasionally sufficient to break bones. This danger has been obviated through the introduction of the use of the drug, curare, in connection with shock treatment. Curare, as you probably know, is the principal active ingredient of the arrow poison used by certain South American aborigines. It has a very curious and sharply localized effect. It puts out of action temporarily the end plates of the motor nerves in the muscles. It is not an anesthetic and has little or no effect upon any other part of the nervous system. Thus, while the electric current produces the same violent reaction in the brain, and the same strong stimuli are sent out over the motor nerves, under the influence of the drug these stimuli are stopped or reduced in the end plates of the motor nerves; and the muscles either do not react or react much less violently, depending upon the dosage of curare.

Shock treatments are usually given every other day in courses of from eight to twenty treatments. While the physiologic or psychologic mechanism of this form of treatment is not clear, the results are beneficial in properly selected cases. Like other new and dramatic forms of treatment, shock treatment has been overexploited in too many instances; but, in the hands of a competent psychiatrist, it is a valuable addition to the treatment of mental illness. It has one effect which, if it did nothing else, would make it worth while. In the usual case, it quiets the disturbed and violent patient, thus simplifying his care and improving his general health. Without electroshock, we would have been hard put to give adequate care to the disturbed psychotic patients in the European Theater of Operations in World War II. Few of our military hospitals in Europe were adequately constructed or equipped to protect violent patients; and the accommodations for such cases on hospital ships and troop transports were so limited that only a few could have been returned safely to the United States. Fortunately, one or two courses of electro-shock so quieted most disturbed patients that they could be properly cared for in Europe and safely transported back to the United States.

One curious fact about the shock treatment of mental illness is that the observation of the German psychiatrist around which the method was developed—the observation that epileptics never develop schizophrenia—was not correct. Epileptics do develop schizophrenia, or, better perhaps, schizophrenics sometimes do have epilepsy. However, it was one of those fortunate mistakes out of which has come great good.

Of much more recent origin than shock therapy is actual cutting surgery upon the brain in cases of mental illness. There are many reasons to believe that the frontal lobes of the brain, lying just above and behind the eyes, are concerned in the mechanism through which the individual becomes integrated in society. Injuries to the frontal lobe are frequently followed by abrupt and profound changes in behavior. One of the most famous of these cases was that in which a crowbar, being used to tamp a charge of blasting powder in a hole in rock, was driven, by accidental explosion of the charge, through the front and top of a man's head, destroying most of his frontal lobes. The victim did not even lose consciousness despite the terrific nature of the injury. He made an uneventful physical recovery, retained a mentality well within what is generally regarded as normal limits, but rapidly developed traits of character quite different from his previous disposition, and was not thereafter nearly so well-adjusted to his environment.

Starting from these few facts, a psychiatrist reasoned that severing the nerve paths from the frontal lobes to the rest of the brain would end or lessen the influence of the frontal lobes upon the behavior of the individual; and that, when this behavior was abnormal because of mental illness, it might be abnormal because of the influence of deranged function of the frontal lobes. If this were true, blocking the influence of the frontal lobes through cutting the paths connecting them with the rest of the brain would at least remove this source of contribution to abnormal behavior. This is the theory upon which the operation known as prefrontal lobotomy was devised.

The operation is relatively simple so far as brain surgery is concerned. In the first operations of this character, an incision was made and a hole drilled through the skull just above the temple. A knife was thrust into the brain toward the nerve paths to be severed, and given a sweep up and down to cut these nerve fibres. A recent refinement of the operation consists in entering the skull at the top, and carefully dissecting down to the fibers to be cut. The field is visible, and the surgeon can see at all times what he is cutting.

This operation is done on both sides of the brain. It is done under local anesthesia, and often a conversation carried on with the patient during the cutting of the nerve fibers is of some assistance in determining the extent of the cutting. The brain, while the seat of all sensation, is itself insensitive to pain.

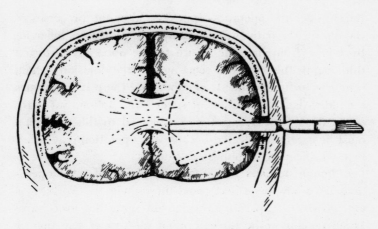

FIG. 12. DIAGRAMMATIC REPRESENTATION OF THE FIRST OPER-
ATION OF PREFRONTAL LOBOTOMY. A KNIFE IS INSERTED
THROUGH A HOLE DRILLED IN THE SIDE OF THE SKULL; AND,
WHEN ITS CUTTING END REACHES THE TRACT TO BE SEVERED,
IT IS SWEPT BACK AND FORTH. AN IDENTICAL OPERATION IS
PERFORMED ON THE OTHER SIDE OF THE HEAD.

From *Psychosurgery*, by W. J. Freeman and J. W. Watts, 1942;
with permission of the authors and by courtesy of Charles C.
Thomas, Publisher, Springfield, Illinois.

Recently, Dr. Walter Freeman has devised a simplified
technique for prefrontal lobotomy. He uses an instrument
very similar to an ordinary ice pick. Anesthetizing the
patient with electroshock, he drives this instrument through
the upper part of the orbit of each eye into the frontal lobes
of the brain; and, by sweeping the point back and forth,
destroys the association paths. In Doctor Freeman's hands
this operation has been very successful; but most neuro-
surgeons prefer the open operation.

The results of prefrontal lobotomy are unpredictable.

Rarely does the operation appear to alter the processes of thought of the patient, but usually it improves his behavior by taking from him the desire to act upon his distorted thinking, or the energy to react against the delusions which formerly tortured him. After lobotomy, there is sometimes a childish lack of restraint of speech and action, but without malice. However, patients subjected to this operation must be carefully selected because the operation may result in intensification of undesirable traits.

Although perhaps 10,000, or even more, of these operations have now been performed throughout the world, it is yet too early to pass final judgment upon the procedure. Much remains to be learned about the proper selection of cases for this treatment. I know of results that can be described as little short of miraculous—people who have been confined for years in institutions, completely out of contact with the world of reality, with the outlook hopeless, and who, after prefrontal lobotomy have been able not only to leave the hospital but to resume important positions in the business or professional world. At the other extreme are cases which seem to be worse after operation. The consensus of current opinion is that the ability of lobotomized patients to resume their former positions in society depends largely upon the demands of that position. It seems to have been convincingly demonstrated that these patients rarely are thereafter able to indulge in abstract thought, or to make sound decisions in complex problems. Rarely would a mathematician, after lobotomy, be able to solve involved equations in higher mathematics; nor could a financier thereafter rely upon his judgment in the stock market. On the other hand, a deckhand on a ferry boat, or a char-

woman, might be expected to return to productive oc-
cupation.

The present conservative estimate of the value of prefrontal lobotomy is that one-third the cases are improved,
one-third are unchanged, and one-third are worsened by
the operation. This evaluation is probably correct insofar
as the mental condition of patients is concerned. However,
the usual result, even in patients who do not recover to the
point of being able to leave the institution, is that, after
operation, they are more tractable and much less difficult
to care for.

Prefrontal lobotomy has been criticized as an empirical
procedure—a shot in the dark with no means of knowing
exactly what is hit, since the path of the knife beneath the
surface of the brain is determined by feel and not by vision.
This criticism does not apply to the refined operative technique. Furthermore, say the critics, nerve paths are cut
indiscriminately—some that perhaps should not be cut as
well as those that should; and, in some cases, a failure to
cut all that should be cut. There is some validity in this
criticism.

More recent research is directed toward a reasoned,
rational selection of the brain areas to be destroyed. The
functions of some, but by no means all, of the areas of
the brain have been established. Research is now directed
toward the removal of definite areas, but it is still difficult
to locate these with accuracy. Two new operations upon
this principle have been devised, but both are still in the
experimental stage. The first of these is one given the name
of thalamotomy. In this operation, the destruction of the
nerve paths is done in the optic thalamus—which is at the
forward end of the brain stem. Areas to be destroyed are

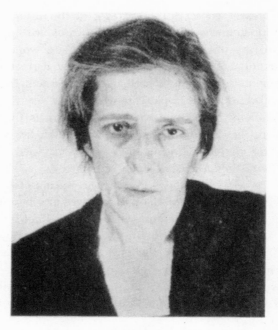

FIG. 13. A PATIENT WITH INVOLUTIONAL
DEPRESSION OF SIX YEARS' DURATION
WITH COMPLETE DISABILITY AND CON-
STANT SUICIDAL IDEAS; BEFORE PRE-
FRONTAL LOBOTOMY.

From *Psychosurgery*, by W. J. Freeman and
J. W. Watts, 1942; with permission of the
authors and by courtesy of Charles C.
Thomas, Publisher, Springfield, Illinois.

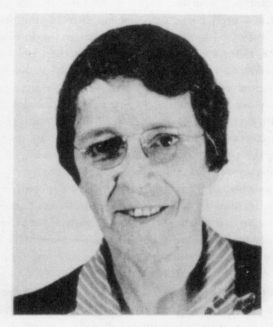

FIG. 14. SAME PATIENT AS SHOWN IN FIG. 13, FIVE WEEKS AFTER PREFRONTAL LOBOTOMY; SHE WAS THEN PLANNING TO RETURN TO HER POSITION.

From *Psychosurgery*, by W. J. Freeman and J. W. Watts, 1942; with permission of the authors and by courtesy of Charles C. Thomas, Publisher, Springfield, Illinois.

first located through knowledge of that part of the thalamus to which many of the fibers from the frontal lobes go. The actual destruction of the nerve centers is done by coagulation with a high frequency electric current—the so-called "radio knife." This minimizes the danger of hemorrhage. Thus far, there appears to be little difference between the result of lobotomy and of thalamotomy—except that convulsive seizures seem to be less frequent after thalamotomy than they are after lobotomy. This may be because there is less brain damage in the operation of thalamotomy. Because of the extremely precise techniques which must be used in locating the nucleus of the thalamus to be destroyed, thalamotomy is a very long and very tedious affair.

Still another surgical approach to this problem is being carefully explored. A number of researchers, one group being made up from the medical faculty of Columbia University and from the staff on the Greystone State Hospital in New Jersey, are experimenting in the total removal of certain previously identified areas in the frontal lobes. They have named this operation "topectomy." It takes a long time to evaluate the results of this kind of treatment with any accuracy. One serious handicap is inability, as yet, to locate with accuracy the areas on the surface of the brain which it is desired to remove.

Prefrontal lobotomy is also coming into use as a method of controlling intractable pain, especially that associated with the terminal stages of incurable disease, such as advanced cancer. Among the principal investigators in this field is Dr. John E. Scarff, of the medical faculty of Columbia University, with whom it was my great pleasure to serve in the European Theater of Operations during World War II. A number of most interesting facts have been unearthed in these investigations. It has been found, for example, that unilateral lobotomy is about as effective for such a purpose as is bilateral lobotomy; and that—which is of great interest—it makes little difference whether the operation be done on the one or the other side of the brain. Although many of the brain functions are centered in the so-called dominant or controlling hemisphere of the brain—the left hemisphere in right-handed people, and vice versa—regardless of this and regardless of the location of the source of the pain, the operation is equally effective when done on one or the other frontal lobe.

Another curious discovery is that patients, who have had to consume huge daily doses of morphine for relief from pain, after lobotomy can often abandon the drug abruptly without the slightest difficulty. This is contrary to all other experience in morphine addiction. The so-called "withdrawal symptoms" that follow the rapid reduction of dosage in the treatment of morphine addiction, are of the most profound character, often more than the patient can stand, and necessitate a very gradual reduction in dosage. Yet here are patients who have been on excessive doses of morphine for some time, and who by every past criterion are confirmed addicts; and who, after unilateral lobotomy, are able to stop the drug abruptly without the slightest discomfort. This experience is unique in the history of drug addiction, and it may well point the way for future research in this field.

Mental illness has been with us for a very long time. Perhaps it was one of the first of man's serious afflictions to be recognized. Until very recently, little progress was made in either prevention or treatment. When MacBeth's physician confessed his impotence in the case of Lady MacBeth's diseased mind, MacBeth gave vent to his disgust by snapping—

Throw physic to the dogs; I'll none of it.

Millions of people, either themselves victims of mental illness throughout the centuries, or friends or relatives of those afflicted, must have felt much as did MacBeth. But, recently, the lamp of hope has begun to burn more brightly, and soon mental illness may be conquered as have infectious diseases and many other of the scourges of man. When this comes to pass, medicine will have made its greatest contribution to mankind. For, as a sixteenth century poet said,

> My mind to me a kingdom is,
> Such present joys therein I find,
> That it excels all other bliss
> That earth affords or grows by kind.[2]

[2] Sir Edward Dyer, 1588.

THE SOCIO-ECONOMIC ASPECTS
OF MEDICAL CARE

PART I

Economic history of medical care. Relationship of increased cost to improvement of quality. Development of public responsibility in field of health and medical care

THE ORIGIN of medical practice is lost in antiquity. No one knows when sick and injured persons began to turn to certain individuals for assistance. Even as there now are some lay individuals who boast of a supernatural ability to cure the sick, there must have appeared early in social organization some who appointed themselves or were appointed by common consent to minister to the sick and injured. Until quite recently, considerable prestige was attached to such a vocation; and the presence of healers is common in even the most primitive societies.

Formal instruction in the healing arts dates only from the sixth or seventh century, B. C., although there seems to have been some instruction in healing in the temples of Saturn some four thousand years before Christ. The ancient Greeks developed the first rational system of medical practice, and they retained a monopoly in it for more than two hundred years.

The early centuries of the Christian era were characterized by attempts to establish rigid rules for the study and practice of the arts and sciences. The church was reducing theology to a more or less empirical discipline; and, since the church was for centuries the seat of all formal learning, the art of medicine was caught in this general pattern of thought.

It was for this reason that there was little advance in medical knowledge from the time that Galen formulated his theories of physiology in the second century, A. D., until Harvey, in the seventeenth century, struck off the shackles that had restrained medical research for almost fifteen centuries. It is true that, during these centuries, a few pertinent observations had been offered which conflicted with Galen's theories; but, for the most part, these were regarded as heretical and untrue only because they would, if accepted, upset the pattern of thought which had become traditional. Even Harvey's convincing demonstration of the circulation of the blood was first received with derision and anger, because it destroyed, at one stroke, the foundation of all medical theory of the day.

Hospitals originated as institutions dedicated exclusively to the medical care of the indigent, and so continued for many centuries. Their development as well-equipped workshops, essential to the best medical and surgical practice, is a matter of not much more than a half-century. In fact, prior to the discovery of the causes and methods of transmission of infection, hospitals were not places of choice in which to be sick. For almost every ailment and injury, the case fatality was considerably higher in hospitals than in private homes. There were several reasons for this. The poor often delayed seeking attention until their ailments were in an advanced stage. Their physical condition was usually substandard, and their resistance thereby lowered. But, more important, the hospital was filled with infection of all kinds; and, since the cause and mode of transmission were not known, infection spread from one case to another. Because of this reputation, hospitals were shunned by all people who could afford to pay at least the minimum fees for medical care in their homes. This had a very important bearing upon the economics of medical care of the time.

Even the great impetus given to surgery by the discovery of anesthesia did not extend, to any degree, the usefulness of hospitals to the self-supporting public. The private home continued to be the place of choice for major surgery as well as for minor illness.

However, the discovery of the causes of infection introduced problems of aseptic technique which could not be solved satisfactorily in the home. Thorough sterilization required too much heavy machinery. Furthermore, now that the dangers of infection were controllable, the field of surgery expanded rapidly, and better aids were required in the way of lighting and plumbing which were difficult to provide in the home. These advances made the hospital a necessary adjunct of good surgery, and altered its character from a charitable institution to an essential workshop. Instead of being the most dangerous place in which to be sick, the hospital became the safest.

Until this time, practically all hospitals were public institutions supported in whole or in part by tax money. Citizens, able to pay for medical care, ordinarily were not eligible for admission. Whether or not public hospitals were available to the self-supporting public, they were not acceptable because of their traditional association with charity, austerity of comforts, and reputation for high mortality.

This new situation created a heavy demand for hospital facilities for people who could afford to pay, in whole or in part, for their care; and voluntary hospitals increased rapidly in number. Whether because of the long association of hospitals with charitable aims, or whether because of the inadequate number of free beds in public institutions, most of the new voluntary hospitals were built with some free ward beds.

It was some years before public funds became available for partial payment for the care of the indigent in the public wards of voluntary hospitals. For many years, this cost was met by voluntary contributions from philanthropic citizens. The annual drive for funds for voluntary hospitals was a fixed affair in the routine of administration. So generous was the usual response to such appeals that there was always money that could be used to pay some part of the cost of caring for paying patients; and underpricing of hospital services for all patients became the rule in voluntary hospital operation. This, too, is a most important factor in the changing economics of medical care.

The next social change which exterted a great influence upon voluntary hospitals was the disappearance of the domestic servant from the homes of people in the middle and low income brackets. Fifty years ago, when maids were paid two to five dollars per week, it was indeed a poor family that could not, and did not, afford at least one house servant. When rising wages, the opening of the doors of business and industry to women, and the attachment of social stigma to domestic service, drove the servants from homes, the care of the sick in the home became considerably more difficult—particularly if the afflicted one was the housewife herself. This new inability to house the sick at home became another important factor in the economics of medical care.

Then, too, as one-family homes became smaller and smaller, and as larger homes were occupied by more families —all the results of inflated building costs and a housing shortage—the care of sick in many homes has become almost an impossibility; and hospitals more and more are being used even for trivial illnesses. This has added to the average cost of medical care.

Finally, recent advances in medical practice have introduced more and more precise techniques which now can only be carried out in well-equipped hospitals. The apparatuses and personnel required are beyond the means of the average physician practicing alone. They are to be had in the larger group clinics; and, as such group practice grows, there will be less necessity for the use of hospitals for the diagnostic work-up of ambulant cases.

So much for the greatly increased use of hospitals in medical care. This, alone, would have added considerably to the cost. But the cost of hospital operation has more than trebled in the last few years. The greatest increase in operating costs has been in the field of labor—professional, skilled and unskilled. Only a few years ago, most personnel in hospitals worked a 60 to 72 hour week. Today, few work more than 44 hours and some as little as 40 hours in a week. The weekly wage has been more than doubled at the same time that the weekly work has been cut almost in half. Furthermore, new techniques and refinement of old ones has made necessary more employee-hours of work per patient-day. The labor cost in hospitals has almost quadrupled in the past fifteen years—certainly it has tripled.

The cost of every item that hospitals must buy—food, fuel, linens, and the rest—has risen greatly, just as the general cost of living has risen. The new antibiotic drugs are more expensive than the old stand-bys and are used in staggering quantities. In one recent survey, made in a representative area, the cost of drugs per patient-day in hospital in 1947 was 4.4 times that of 1938.

At the same time that hospitals were faced with spiralling costs of operation, one large source of their revenue was being rapidly obliterated. This was the voluntary contributions from charitable citizens. Heavy taxation has almost completely dried up the sources of private philanthropy. The Socialists regard this as a great blessing; but of that I am not so sure. In so doing, we have robbed our people of great spiritual values that can never be replaced unless and until we change this situation. When an individual contributes to a worthy cause, both he and the beneficiary benefit. It is a blessing to be able to give; and the giver thereby gains spiritual values. But, when money for welfare is taken forcibly by taxation, the individual citizen feels no responsibility for the causes for which it is to be spent. When all welfare is supported by tax money, our citizens will no longer feel any personal responsibility for their less fortunate brethren. This is a paradoxical and a tragic product of the Welfare State.

In any event, this withdrawal of voluntary support of hospitals has added greatly to their difficulties. This loose money now goes for taxes, but little tax money goes to voluntary hospitals. In most cases, the government—local, state or Federal—pays niggardly rates for the care of public charges by voluntary hospitals; and so these hospitals lose money on every patient cared for as a public charge.

Coincident with the depletion of the wells of private philanthropy, the returns from the investment of endowment funds have sunk to an all-time low, because of a lowering of interest rates by the deficit financing of the Federal Government. So, now we seem about to be caught in a vicious circle. The cost of medical care has become burdensome, largely because of a change in our political philosophy which occurred some fifteen years ago. Having created the situation, some of our politicians now advance it as an impelling reason for pushing still farther into the Welfare State. It seems not to have occurred to these leftist lawmakers that the wisdom of retracing some of our steps toward national socialism might well be explored.

So, to summarize the present difficulty of hospitals, operating costs have risen greatly and sources of revenue have been reduced virtually to one—the patient himself. Since patients must now largely pay the entire cost of hospital operation, and this in an inflated market, it is little wonder that payment of hospital bills is beyond the ability of many.

But, worse than that, the poor patient is forced to pay for a lot of services not directly connected with his own stay in the hospital. Almost every hospital operates one or more public services at a heavy loss. Among these are the emergency room for accident cases, the ambulance service, the school of nursing, and the training of interns and residents. There was a time when schools of nursing and resident training were sources of cheap professional labor and were assets to the hospital. Those days are gone forever. Elevation of educational standards and the increased cost of maintenance has made teaching in hospitals a financial liability, regardless of its importance in patient care and as a public service. But it is not fair that the patient in the hospital carry his burden in whole or in large part. Government thus far has shown no eagerness to assume this responsibility, which is a public responsibility just as is any other kind of education; and we are now witnessing our Government level attacks against the cost of voluntary medical care when a significant part of that cost is the result of the failure of the Government to discharge its own responsibility.

Thus far we have developed that part of the cost of medical care which is associated with hospitals—the rapid increase in the use of hospitals and the inflated cost of hospital operation. What about the doctor cost?

Insofar as the individual fees of physicians and surgeons are concerned, they have failed to keep abreast of the general rise in living costs. Countrywide, doctors' fees have increased only about 30 to 35 percent during the time that the cost of living has gone up more than 70 percent. Today there are more appendixes removed for $100, or even less, than there are for fees larger than that—and $100 was the standard fee for an appendectomy among people of moderate means when I was a boy. The charges of individual doctors have added very little to the increasing cost of medical care.

But modern medical care requires more doctors and more allied personnel in the health field than did the medical care of even twenty-five years ago. Except in cases of little consequence, no longer is one doctor adequate with all his diagnostic and therapeutic equipment in a little black bag. There are X-rays to be taken, blood chemistries to be done, basal metabolism tests to be made. The scope of medical knowledge has become so wide that no longer can one physician or surgeon feel competent in a very broad field; and, in justice to the patient, he must have consultation far more frequently than did his professional grandfather.

The increased cost of doctor services is to be found largely in the field of diagnosis rather than in the field of treatment. As has been pointed out, individual fees have risen only slightly; and, once the diagnosis has been established, it does not take much more medical manpower to treat a case, even with involved surgery, than it did twenty-five years ago. But it does require more medical and allied manpower to make a diagnosis. This is more costly, but it is infinitely more accurate. Any saving in cost in this direction would be the poorest kind of economy.

I do not see where there can be any reduction in the comparative cost of medical care without lowering of quality. Of course, if costs in general go down, the cost of medical care will drop accordingly. This will be true especially of the hospital fraction of the cost of medical care. But it is quite possible that new discoveries and greater refinement of techniques may bring additional cost.

The present cost of medical care is a serious matter—one which worries more of us than the present consumers. It would be alarming were there not a way to meet it without too great hardship. Medical care is the one human necessity the cost of which cannot be predicted in advance. Even in times of rising costs, the cost of food, of clothing, of shelter, and of all other necessities can be predicted for some weeks in advance. The costs of these necessities are easy to budget. But no one can predict how much medical care he will need next week, or what it will cost.

However unpredictable this may be in the individual case, like many other risks in life it is predictable in the group. So, the cost of medical care is an insurable risk. So long as the cost of medical care was relatively low, no one was interested in insuring against it. There was never much point in insuring a bicycle, but the automobile is a different risk.

Nevertheless, the prepayment of medical costs long antedates the time when they became unduly burdensome. So far as we have been able to find, the earliest health prepayment plan on the North American continent was one established in the year 1655 at Ville-Marie on the Island of Montreal. According to a document dated March 3 of that year: "Urbain Tessier, dit Lavigne, and 36 others, acting both for themselves and their families and children, contracted with Etienne Bouchard, Master Surgeon of the said Ville-Marie, for the latter to dress and to physic all sorts of illness, whether natural or accidental, except the plague of small-pox, leprosy, epilepsy and lithotomy, or cutting for the stone, in consideration of the sum of 100 sous each year, payable by each of the above-mentioned persons, in two terms and quarters, and to treat also their children who may hereafter be born." This contract was cancellable by either party "upon giving notice to those concerned, such notice to avail only for the years which have not yet begun to run."

This contract of three hundred years ago contained the principal elements of a present-day health insurance contract. It named the subscribers, listed the benefits, set forth clearly the exclusions, and provided for cancellation by either party.

A few years later, in 1681 and likewise in Montreal, the Rev. Mother Renée le Jumeau, Superior of the Dames Religieuses Hospitalières, contracted with Sieur Jean Martinent de Fonblanche and with Antoine Forestier, both Master Surgeons, for medical and surgical services for patients in the sisters' hospital, "in consideration of the sum of 75 livres each for each year, and upon the condition that the said Surgeons, cannot claim or seek to recover anything else whatever from the said patients." Here is established the principle of the full-service contract.

The system of prepayment of the costs of medical care seems to have been devised, fostered, and developed by the Roman Catholic Church. We have just mentioned two very early projects. During the lumbering days of the late 1870's and 1880's in Northern Michigan and Minnesota, there was little provision for the medical care of lumberjacks. At the same time, Catholic sisters in that part of the United States were having a hard time finding the necessary funds to keep their little hospitals going. The problems of each party were solved by a happy idea of the sisters. They visited each lumber camp each month and sold what was called a "hospital ticket" for a dollar each. This ticket entitled the holder to care in one of the sisters' hospitals. At first glance, considering the low costs of the day, hospital care insurance at a dollar a month for the single subscriber must have been a profitable business for these enterprising sisters. That rate is not far out of line with present-day costs. However, the accident rate was probably high, and, for other reasons, lumberjacks were probably not preferred risks. In any event, the little sisters kept the business going so long as lumbering operations were continued on a large scale, and other sisters began similar plans when the lumber industry moved westward. We can be certain that these clever and devoted women did not lose money; and we can be sure that any excessive profits were spent in a good cause. There were no insurance commissioners to worry them.

In 1912, a plan for the prepayment of hospital costs was organized in Rockford, Illinois, under the name of the

Rockford Association. In 1921, one hospital in Grinnell, Iowa, developed a plan covering cost of room and board and nursing, in that hospital, up to a period of three weeks. No ancillary hospital service was included. The Thompson Benefit Association for hospital service was organized in Brattleboro, Vermont, in 1927. This plan also covered the fees of the surgeon, but had a maximum limit of all benefits of $300.

The plan, however, which is generally considered to be the prototype of present Blue Cross Plans is that organized in 1929 by the schoolteachers of Dallas, Texas. This plan was developed in connection with the Baylor University Hospital and through the cooperation of Dr. Judson Ford Kimball, then the Vice-President of the University. Approximately 1,500 teachers were insured against the cost of hospital care at the rate of $6.00 per person per year. The benefits included not only room and board and nursing, but also the use of the operating room, laboratory, and anesthesiology fees, and routine medication and dressings. Full coverage was provided for a maximum of 21 days, with a 33 percent discount upon charges for stays in excess of three weeks. Shortly after the plan was started, enrollment privilege was extended to other people than schoolteachers.

From this single Plan with its initial 1,500 subscribers, Blue Cross has grown, in 20 years, to 90 approved Plans with approximately 36 million subscribers. As of 31 December 1948, 21.3 percent of the people in the United States are protected by Blue Cross. At the rate at which Blue Cross is now growing, it is probable that, as of this evening, approximately 23 percent of our people have Blue Cross protection.

This enrollment is not spread evenly throughout the

country. In Rhode Island, for example, 73 percent of the population are in Blue Cross; in Delaware, 54 percent; in Connecticut, 43 percent; and, in New York, 37 percent. This week, Associated Hospital Service of New York (the Blue Cross Plan in this metropolitan area) celebrates the enrollment of its four millionth member. These Plans have been in existence longer than many in the South and West, but the latter are growing very fast. Maryland and Missouri each have about 30 percent of their population, and Michigan and Illinois about 25 percent.

While to the purveyors of health care, hospital service and the services of physicians and surgeons are two separate and distinct operations, the public makes no such distinction. To the man on the street, it is all the cost of sickness. For this reason, Blue Cross cannot fill the whole need for protection against the costs of medical care.

Aside from the pioneering in this field in Montreal in the seventeenth century, mentioned before, the first medical care plan, which can be described as a community enterprise, seems to have been one initiated at the turn of the last century in Tampa, Florida. It was organized largely among the Cuban cigarmakers, not only to provide medical and hospital care but also for purposes of general welfare. It was named "Centro Español de Tampa," and is still in existence. Its revenues are derived both from subscriptions of members and from social activities. Medical care is furnished subscribers by a panel of salaried physicians.

The first large area in which medical care plans developed was the Pacific Northwest. Certain abuses developed out of sharp competition; and, as early as 1917, county medical societies began to take a hand in the management to stop these abuses. County medical service bureaus were established which contracted with employers for the medical care of employees, permitting the latter to have a free choice of participating physicians. In the State of Washington, these plans continue as county medical bureaus, there being now 22 such bureaus operating in that State. In Oregon, almost all of the county bureaus have merged into a state plan under the name of Oregon Physicians' Service.

The first state-wide plan to be organized was California Physicians' Service, started in 1939 by the California State Medical Association. In 1945, a national federation of medical care plans was organized under the name of Associated Medical Care Plans and with the Blue Shield as the symbol of approved plans. There are now 60 Blue Shield Plans in the United States with a total enrollment of more than eleven million.

Forty-seven Blue Shield Plans are joined in a cooperative working agreement with 56 Blue Cross Plans in offering the public both medical and hospital care in a single package. The difference in numbers of the Plans so joined is due to the different territorial limits of Blue Cross and Blue Shield Plans. One Blue Shield Plan may cover territory divided between two or more Blue Cross Plans. Blue Shield Plans, associated with Blue Cross Plans, are growing at a much faster rate than those operating alone—which is added evidence that the public wants full protection in one package.

The rapid growth of the two voluntary nonprofit agencies, Blue Cross and Blue Shield, sometimes makes us forget that there are many other agencies in the United States offering similar or comparable protection. The ninety-odd insurance companies offering health and accident insurance have some thirty-five million policies in effect. Some of these are exclusively accident policies; and a conservative estimate of the number of people protected by commerical carriers against the costs of medical care is twenty million.

Then there are the cooperatives which include a few million more. There are 18 million veterans who, for all practical purposes, even if it is questionable whether this is the intent of the law, are entitled to medical and hospital care at Government expense. Many of these have other protection, so they cannot be added in as a separate group. Six and one-half million workers are protected by workmen's compensation insurance. The Armed Forces, totalling with dependents almost three million, are provided medical and hospital care.

Adding all these groups together and subtracting a liberal figure for any duplications, a very conservative estimate of the number of people in this country who are protected in full or in large part against the costs of medical and hospital care is about sixty million. The number who are too indigent to pay for such protection, or who are uninsurable, has been estimated to be twenty million. These have always been public charges, or have been furnished medical care free by public or voluntary hospitals and the medical profession—medical care, I might add, of the highest quality.

The estimates are most conservative. Some informed individuals have estimated that the number of people protected to a significant degree by one or another plan is in excess of ninety million. I have used the figure of sixty million.

In any event, at the rate at which all of these plans are growing, it will not be long before 100 million of our people have protection. As to how many need such protection, the estimates range all the way from 75 to 120 million. Personally, I feel that coverage of 80 million will fulfill every real need.

At present, the protection against the costs of medical and hospital care falls into three general types of plans. All three types have a few characteristics in common, although they differ widely in other respects. All place more or less limitation upon the length of time that they will protect against one attack of the same illness. None will continue protection for indefinite periods in such long-duration illnesses as tuberculosis, mental diseases, and the chronic infirmities of old age, although all do provide coverage of these afflictions for a limited period.

All three types place some limitation upon eligibility for benefits in preexisting conditions, such as requiring a reasonable waiting period before the beneficiary becomes eligible for maternity benefits and for such surgical operations of election as the repair of preexisting hernias and the removal of tonsils and adenoids. The necessity for such protection against abuses is obvious.

The three general types of prepayment plans can further be classified into those which provide medical care exclusively or largely through agencies under their own control, and those which permit the beneficiary to select his own physician and hospital.

The cooperative type of medical plan is one which usually provides the greater part of the medical care through clinics and/or hospitals which the agency, itself, operates. These cooperatives are sponsored by farm organizations, labor unions, associations of government employees, and, in a few cases, by special organizations created for this specific purpose.

Each of these cooperatives operates its own clinic, and a few, in addition, operate their own hospitals. Most employ their staffs, both professional and lay, on a full-time basis with fixed salary schedules, although at least one operates under an arrangement whereby a part-time professional staff divides among the participating physicians a part of the income of the plan.

These cooperatives are among the oldest of the plans for the prepayment of the costs of medical care, yet they have grown least of all. The reason for this slow growth appears to be that they are not very popular either with physicians or with subscribers.

Those which operate with full-time staffs upon fixed salaries are unattractive to the great majority of physicians for the reasons that their very terms of employment do not permit of time to be spent in teaching and in other similar pursuits by which most physicians like to keep abreast of the advances in their profession. It is true that there are many great physicians who are employed upon straight salaries; but the vast majority of these are employed by medical schools and teaching hospitals where the opportunities for professional advancement and improvement have a far greater appeal than money. These opportunities are rarely open to the full-time employees of cooperative medical plans, so that the principle inducement is the salary they are paid—not a very heavy inducement to most of us who entered medicine.

From the side of the patient, most people do not like the pattern of medical practice which the cooperatives are compelled, in the interest of efficient administration, to adopt. Obviously, choice of physicians is limited to those employed by the cooperative and, in the case of a specialist, to those with whom the cooperative has a working agreement. But ordinarily choice is still further restricted, and the beneficiary must accept the service of whatever clinic physician happens to be unoccupied at the moment. This often results in the patient seeing a different physician upon successive visits to the clinic for the same illness. A friend of mine, who is a subscriber to one of these cooperative plans, was ill last winter—confined to bed in his home. Three different doctors from the clinic visited him on three successive days. He had never seen any of them before, upon his visits to the clinic. By the end of the third day, he became discouraged and decided to call off his own illness.

A second type of plan for the prepayment of medical and hospital costs is that offered by a number of commercial insurance companies. This is very similar to other types of insurance we have known for many years in many fields of risk, such as protection against losses by fire, losses at sea, and against the hazards of owning and operating an automobile. In consideration of a premium paid at intervals by the insured person, the insurance company agrees to pay him a specified number of dollars in the event of certain prescribed events in the field of his health. For example, such a policy provides for payment to the policyholder of a specified amount of money for each day he is required to spend in a hospital and/or for each medical or surgical attention he receives, not to exceed the over-all limit fixed in the policy.

This type of insurance is known as indemnity insurance, since it indemnifies the policyholder with money for the losses he incurs through the necessity for medical care. The insurance company pays the money, in the amount fixed by the policy, directly to the policyholder, regardless of whether his hospital or doctor bills are greater or less than the amount of the indemnity.

The amount of the indemnity varies in more or less direct relation to the premium charged, or vice versa. Many different policies, with different benefits and different premiums, are offered by insurance companies. Obviously, the lower the cost, the lower the benefits.

Policies of this kind, that are offered by the sound, ethical insurance companies, give fair value to the policyholder. But, before he purchases this type of policy, the citizen should assure himself that he is dealing with a reputable and ethical company, because there are too many wholly unscrupulous companies in this business, whose policies provide, in very fine print not often read by the policyholder until his claim is denied, a long list of exclusions and of conditions under which payment will be made.

Many people prefer this type of protection. Its principal advantages are that it guarantees the premium rate for a period usually as long as one year, and since payment is made to the policyholder rather than to the hospital or doctor, he is free to use the money as he may elect. Others do not choose indemnity insurance as a protection against the cost of medical care, principally because its benefits are a fixed indemnity. In a period of rising costs, benefits of $10.00 per day may cover hospital costs one year, but pay no more than half to two-thirds of the costs the next year. Furthermore, in the case of people of low-income, the doctor has not obligated himself to charge no more for his services than the amount of indemnity paid.

A third type of prepayment plan is that offering what is known as a service contract. A service contract differs from an indemnity contract in that it provides for the payment of hospital and doctor bills regardless of the amount, whereas an indemnity contract provides for the payment of a certain amount of money regardless of what the hospital and doctor bills may be. Payments made under a service contract are made directly to the hospitals and doctors—never to the subscriber. Thus, the subscriber receives services instead of being paid in dollars.

Service contracts are written almost exclusively by the two great voluntary nonprofit Plans—Blue Cross for hospital costs, and Blue Shield for doctor's bills.

So, people now have the choice among three different types of protection against the costs of medical and hospital care. With the exception of the fraudulent indemnity contracts sold by certain unethical companies, the citizen obtains value received from each type. One thing he must remember—the more protection he gets, the more must he pay for it.

The traditional policy of both Blue Cross and Blue Shield is to offer as much protection as can be priced within the reach of the lowest-income self-supporting groups. They could, without difficulty, extend their protection to cover almost every conceivable contingency in health care; but to do so would restrict their market to the well-to-do, and this would defeat their purpose. The other types of prepayment are prepared to meet the demand for high-cost protection, and Blue Cross and Blue Shield will continue a policy of providing the maximum amount of protection compatible with a cost within the reach of almost every self-supporting person and family.

PART II

*Development of the prepayment principle in medical care and
its influence upon the general health. Extension of this
principle to Government compulsory insurance*

Iɴ ᴛʀᴀᴄɪɴɢ the origin of the problems of the economics of
medical care, we have found their principal source to be
the great improvement in the quality of medical care. This
is a most important fact, and one which should be kept
uppermost in our minds as we search for solutions of these
problems.

That increased efficiency is accompanied by increased
cost, while by no means an invariable rule, is still a common experience in our everyday life. Travel by horse and
wagon required a greater outlay of money than did making
a journey afoot. The automobile is more expensive to build
and to operate than a horse-drawn vehicle. The airplane
is still more costly.

It is true that increased production of innovations lowers
the initial cost. It is also true that occasionally mass production makes possible the pricing of an improved article
below that of its inferior predecessor; but this is true only
when machines can be substituted for human brains and
hands.

It would be an untruth if I were to tell you that I shall
present this question of the economics of medical care with
complete objectivity. I wish I were able to do this. But, for
some years, I have been too close to the problem of improving the *quality* of medical care to disregard this essential

element in a search for the solution of the economic problems of medical care.

It has fallen to my lot to have been responsible for the medical care of millions of Americans. Despite any mistakes I have made in the discharge of this responsibility—and I have made mistakes—I have never accepted any other yardstick than quality for the measurement of achievement, nor have I ever confused *quantity* with *quality*. It is vastly more important, for the present as well as for the future, that 80 percent of our people be given medical care of high quality than that 100 percent of our people receive third-rate medical care. If we adhere firmly to quality as the essential criterion, we can extend its benefits to all of our people; but, once we abandon this criterion, we can never again reestablish it.

I realize that the charge may be leveled against me that my want of objectivity arises from a selfish interest in the outcome of this issue between compulsory and voluntary health insurance. Such a charge would be without foundation. It is true that I am, at this moment, connected with the voluntary health insurance movement, but I have no intention of continuing this connection even so long as would be required to place a compulsory insurance scheme in operation if the legislation were passed in this Congress; nor do I intend ever again to engage in any enterprise in the health field. I have, for several years, promised myself to retire from hard work, and to enjoy whatever time remains in the leisurely pursuit of some unprofitable avocation.

For these reasons, it cannot make any difference to me, as an individual, whether this issue is decided one way or another. I have no personal stake in the controversy. I cannot, however, dismiss so casually my concern over the future of medical progress in this country.

The proponents of compulsory health insurance allege that 80 percent of our people are financially unable to afford necessary medical care. In support of this contention, they delight to quote a similar statement attributed to a medical organization some years back. So far as I am concerned, these sources are equally unreliable. One discouraging thing about the matter is that so few facts are known about it; this has operated to remove all limits upon the statements that are made both pro and con. If there were no other reason for postponing hasty action upon such an important innovation in government, this paucity of factual information should caution us against making a leap in the dark.

It is not difficult to show the absurdity of the statement that 80 percent of our people cannot afford the cost of medical care. If this were true, we would have no automotive industry worthy of the name, and no great industries producing radio and television instruments, electric refrigerators and motion pictures. It takes far more than 20 percent of our population to furnish markets for these products. These are largely luxury goods, and the cost of many of them, year after year, is greater than the cost of medical care.

Why, then, are luxury goods within the reach of such a large proportion of our population? The principal reason is that the full cost of few of such items must be paid in one lump sum. Motion pictures and liquor and tobacco are bought in small quantities at regular intervals; and expensive durable goods are paid for in small installments over an extended period.

One difficulty in meeting the costs of medical care

through such individually controlled budgeting is the un-predictability of the need. If medical care were a regularly recurring item, such as the desire for tobacco or the movies, these problems would never have risen—because the amount of money spent in the average family for luxuries would pay many times over for complete medical care.

If it were possible to apply the installment principle to the payment of medical care, this would solve the problem. This is impossible as a complete answer, although it is applied in many cases, for the reason that there is nothing tangible in medical care to serve as collateral against the payment of the debt. If installments are not met upon furniture or automobiles, the article can be recovered to satisfy the unpaid amount. But medical care is a service which must be furnished, usually within a short period, when it is needed. Once furnished, there is nothing tangible upon which to recover; and the more unpaid bills experi-enced, the higher would have to be the charges to paying patients. It is for this reason that prepayment, upon the insurance principle, offers the only successful solution.

What is "the insurance principle?" There are many principles in insurance, but the basic principle is that the premium, or the rate charged for the protection, must bear a direct relation to the risk involved, and must be sufficient in amount both to pay all losses and to cover the cost of administration. The risk involved may and does vary with the individual protected, just as one building may be a greater fire hazard than another building. Such inequalities in risks are compensated for in one of two ways—either by charging a larger or smaller rate for the protection, or by equalizing the average risk by insuring at one time a number of risks. Almost all health insurance operates upon this group insurance principle. By accepting an established group at one time—such as the employees of one industrial plant or the membership of an organization—both good and bad risks are taken. Experience shows the proportion of good and bad risks in any representative group, and the average losses per individual. So, by averaging the expected losses, a flat individual rate can be quoted. This rate will be insufficient to cover the losses incurred by some individuals, and more than sufficient to cover the losses of the others; but it will cover the average loss.

Voluntary health insurance is also available to individuals who are not members of groups. The rates charged are usually fixed—that is, individual variation in risk is not considered—but the insurance plan protects itself against adverse selection in one of three ways. It may charge, for individual protection, a higher rate than for the protection of the individual in the group. It may enroll individuals only in large groups, such as by a community enrollment drive within a limited period—thus making a group from individual members of the community; or it may protect itself against heavy losses by requiring waiting periods before certain benefits become effective. As an example of the last, it is common practice in health insurance to delay maternity benefits until ten months after the enrollment of a family. This protects the plan against the adverse selection of those families which, having knowledge of the existence of pregnancy, would seek protection against the costs of delivery of a child.

It will be evident that, regardless of the method employed to protect a voluntary insurance plan against adverse selection, the rate charged, whether to the individual or to the group, is in relation to the risk involved.

So-called compulsory health insurance operates upon an entirely different principle. The rate charged for the protection bears absolutely no relation to the risk involved. It is based entirely upon the income of the individual protected. Those below a certain level of income pay nothing for their protection. Those in the higher income bracket pay heavily for their protection—actually much more than the protection is worth and much more than they would pay to a voluntary plan for the same amount of protection.

Insofar as the United States is concerned, this is a new principle of insurance; and is not, as Federal Security Administrator Ewing says it is, "the same kind of insurance that has been part of our national fabric for generations."

On the other hand, it is the purest kind of socialism. I hasten to add that I am not damning it for that reason. I am not saying whether socialism is good or bad. If the majority of our people want socialism, if they want our Government to be changed so that we shall become a Welfare State, by all means let us go about it at once; but let us do it with our eyes open and not be deceived as to what we are doing.

One aspect of this issue, which is of minor importance, is its cost. The scope of the medical service to be provided by compulsory health insurance includes complete medical and hospital care for all illnesses, so-called preventive medical care with periodic physical examinations, some dental care, and some drugs and medicines. The wording of the bill is vague in places, perhaps purposely so because it is almost impossible to spell out the benefits under such an inclusive program.

There are several methods by which the cost of compulsory health insurance can be, and has been, estimated. The starting point of one is the cost of protection against the costs of serious illnesses by voluntary health insurance. This varies slightly among the different parts of the country, but the national average is between $30 and $36 per individual per year. Proponents of compulsory health insurance charge that this amount of protection covers only one-third the cost of complete medical care.

Starting with the known cost of the medical care program now in operation in Great Britain, and applying suitable factors for the difference in size of the two populations and for the differences in medical and hospital fees, we arrive again at the surprisingly comparable figure of $100 per capita per annum.

Other approaches to the problem have been made by experienced economists, working independently. All of the results are right at, or very near—some a little below, some a little above—this figure of $100 per person per year. You may remember that, in recent testimony before Congressional Committees, officials of the Federal Security Administration placed the cost of the program they were advocating as "very high," but declined to state any definite figure.

One figure the Federal Security Administration does give. This is that the total income of the compulsory health insurance scheme from payroll deductions and employer contributions, when the program is in full operation, will be $6 billion per annum. At that time, the total cost of the program will be $15 billion per annum, if our entire population is included.

This is an annual deficit of some $9 billion. How is this to be met? It can be met only from the general revenues of the Government. Assuming that aid to Europe will have ceased by that time, this $9 billion will represent an addition of from 20 to 25 percent of the amount of money that must be collected each year through taxes. With a national debt around $250 billion—which must either be paid or repudiated—I wonder whether our Government can assume this heavy additional financial burden and remain solvent. Once the credit of the Government is shaken, the resultant misery and hardship that will come to the low-income citizens will far outweigh any deficiencies in medical care. This fixed charge at $9 billion per year will not decrease in a depression. On the other hand, it will increase because, by reason of unemployment, the payroll deductions and employer contributions will fall off greatly, and all deficits from such contributions must be made up from the general revenues of the Government.

At the same time, the revenues of the Government will shrink—they may fall off as much as 50 percent—and this heavy, fixed charge may well bankrupt the nation.

As I stated before, I consider cost to be of less importance than other factors. But I am unable to see how cost can be wholly disregarded; and I believe that our people should ponder this point well before deciding to accept the principle of compulsory health insurance. Will we get value received? Will we get $9 to $10 billion worth of better health each year? If so, and we have that astronomical amount of money to invest in it, it will be a sound investment. But we cannot disregard those "ifs."

Will compulsory health insurance improve the nation's health? In searching for the answer to that question, let us assay exactly what it will do and what it cannot do.

First, compulsory health insurance will greatly increase

the demand for medical attention. This has been the experience in Great Britain and in every other country in which it has been tried. If the experience in other countries holds good here, this increase will be at least 50 percent, and may be 100 percent. Some part of this increased demand will be furnished by cases in real need of medical care; but the experience elsewhere has been that the large part is made up of cases of little or no consequence, for which medical care would never have been sought formerly.

Whatever may be the moral aspects of occupying the time of doctors and hospitals unnecessarily when the Government is paying the bill instead of the patient, it is not, and can never be made, a violation of law. It is impossible to prevent such abuses. No *true* insurance can survive under such conditions. There would be no fire insurance today if there were no laws against arson—if, at any time a property owner, who was short of ready cash at the moment, could set a match to some insured property and collect the insurance. All insurance *must* be protected against abuses in order to exist.

Here again, the abuse of medical care insurance would not be such a serious matter if increased cost was the only penalty to be paid. There is a much more serious penalty, and one that cannot be calculated in terms of money.

There are only so many doctors and hospitals in this country, so many dentists and nurses, so many medical aides and technicians. Everyone, including the proponents of compulsory health insurance, agrees that there are barely enough medical care facilities and personnel to handle the present demand for medical care. It requires no gigantic intellect to foresee what will happen when the same quantity of facilities must accept a greatly increased load.

It is inevitable that the time devoted to each case must be proportionately decreased, and the thoroughness of the care proportionately lessened. There can be no other result. This is exactly what is happening in Great Britain today. Regardless of whether Americans, who have observed the working of the British scheme at first hand, approve or disapprove of it, they all agree that doctors' offices are overcrowded, that the individual patient receives scant attention, and that patients, in serious need of surgery, must wait long periods before they can be admitted to a hospital. The proponents of compulsory health insurance profess to see in this situation no cause for alarm. This blindness to reality is but a measure of their ignorance of the elements which make up medical care of accepted quality. To them, medical *attention* and medical *care* are synonymous. To the conscientious physician, these are quite different services. The patient, who goes to see his physician and says, "Doctor, I have the itch," and forthwith is given a prescription for an ointment to relieve itching, is being given medical attention; but the patient who consults a physician for the same complaint, is given a thorough examination and discovered to be suffering from diabetes, which is the cause of his itch, is being given medical care.

Lots of medical attention and little medical care is exactly what the people are getting today in Great Britain. A number of observers have reported upon the situation. In order to avoid bias as much as I can, I shall quote from the report of Mr. Lester Velie, which appeared in *Colliers' Magazine* in the issues of March 5 and 12 of this year. Mr. Velie is a champion of compulsory health insurance. The day before these lectures began, I debated the question with him in a public forum in Cincinnati, so that there is no question as to his position. For this reason, I consider his testimony peculiarly competent.

Mr. Velie states that many people in Great Britain, who are now obtaining spectacles, false teeth, wigs and other such accessories without direct payment, and who, in some instances, are able to barter medicinal prescriptions for cosmetics and other toilet preparations, are wholeheartedly in favor of this innovation. This is understandable.

But now I shall quote Mr. Velie directly: "To enter London's great Westminister Hospital for a tonsillectomy, a school child must wait, on the average, fifteen months. A woman requiring urgent [and "urgent" is the word Mr. Velie uses] gynecological surgery must wait seven weeks. So jammed are the free hospitals that many families, even those in modest circumstances, prefer to *pay* the high cost of childbearing . . . rather than take their chances in state institutions."

Mr. Velie then offers his diary of a day spent with a British physician, and I shall quote directly from it. Within 10 minutes after the doctor's waiting room had been opened in the morning, there were some 20 patients gathered. "Against the wall," writes Mr. Velie, "was a queue of boys, clutching prescription forms in one hand and comic books in another." The doctor explained that these boys were following the system which he had had to devise to cope with the daily rush of patients.

As soon as he was ready to begin his morning's work, the doctor opened the door between his consulting room and the waiting room. The first boy in the queue shot his arm through the open door, waving a prescription form. The doctor filled out the form and returned it to the boy. The next boy shot his arm in. "Father's tablets," he announced.

This prescription was written. This procedure was continued until these patients by proxy were served. No patient seen in person, only prescriptions filled out, sight unseen. The next order of business was to see the patients who had called in person. Mr. Velie described only one of these consultations, and I shall give his description. The patient was a workingman with a badly swollen hand. Now I shall quote Mr. Velie directly: "[The doctor] diagnosed the swelling as an infection, prescribed dressings, tonic, rest. 'You'll need several chits, won't you?' asked [the doctor], filling out government prescription form C-10 for free supplies and another slip for sickness benefits. 'How about my eyes, Doctor?' [asked the patient]. . . . The doctor whipped off a green form. He worked unhurriedly, but the patient, forms and all, was disposed of in seven minutes."

This is a colossal irony which seems to have been unconscious on the part of Mr. Velie. Here is a workingman with an infected hand. As every physician knows, the danger of an infected hand is by no means limited to a threat to health and life. Unless carefully and properly treated, such infections are prone to leave the patient with a permanently stiff hand; and, to a workingman, useful hands are essential to his earning his livelihood.

So, here is a patient with a condition which is a potential threat to his future security. He applies for medical care, not only for that but also for his eyes. In the consultation lasting only seven minutes, he gets not only these diagnoses but also three government forms properly filled out. I am quite familiar with the forms devised by the British Government. They are just as involved, just as stupid, and just as useless, as those used by our own Government. No man alive can fill out three of them in less than six minutes and

50 seconds. This left 10 seconds for professional attention to the patient as distinguished from the clerical duties demanded of the physician.

Mr. Velie is again unconsciously ironical. He wrote that the patient was "disposed of" in seven minutes. "Disposed of" seems to be the proper term for the attention given the patient; he was certainly not given medical care. The important lesson of this experience is that all other considerations were subordinated to the "system" which the doctor had had to devise to cope with the demand for attention. This is inevitable in all kinds of government operation. Conformity to a system, abject devotion to forms and to regulations, are placed above all human considerations.

The afternoon of this day of observation of the practice of medicine under compulsory health insurance was devoted to house calls. Mr. Velie says that the doctor made more than a dozen such visits in two hours. This is an average of one house visit in less than ten minutes, including travel time. Mr. Velie does explain that the doctor "strides in and out of patients' homes on the double." I consider that one of the great masterpieces of understatement. Even the most relentless double-time that I ever witnessed in thirty years in the Army could not approach that speed. The only comparable technique of the healing art of which I can think is the absent treatment offered by our Christian Science friends.

Now you might think that this is an unusual case—that this was an incompetent and indifferent physician. Mr. Velie goes to some length to assure us that this is not so. This is one of the better physicians in the city, one whose years of private practice before compulsory health insurance had won for him the confidence and respect of the community. Even if the mockery of this kind of medical practice escaped Mr. Velie, as it seems to have done, apparently the physician labored under no delusion. He told Mr. Velie that he tried not to think what would happen if there were a run of illness later in the winter. I go one step farther—I try not to think what is happening to those patients in the slack season.

A few months ago, one of the most ardent proponents of compulsory health insurance in this country asked one of his acquaintances in London—a gentleman of long experience and distinguished record in the hospital field—how the British scheme was working out in practice. I shall quote directly from the reply to this inquiry: "Now to carry out my promise to give you some information about the working of the new Health Service. Officially it is said to be working well; unofficially it is known that all is not well. . . . The first thing that happened when the Act came into operation . . . was a rush by the public to obtain the services which the Act laid down. But these just did not exist." Here I shall pause to say that this is exactly the same situation that now obtains in this country. Our medical facilities are barely able to meet the present demand. No matter how much more medical care the politicians may promise, it simply cannot be produced at this time, nor for some years to come. To increase the number of hospitals and doctors will require years of time and billions of dollars. To assure the public that compulsory health insurance will solve *this* problem is evidence either of ignorance or of fraud.

This gentleman goes on to say that, as a result of overwork, doctors and nurses are irritable and snap at each other and at patients; that long delays in hospital administration are encountered because decisions have to be made in London rather than by local management; and that the cost is far exceeding the initial estimates. But, to me, the most damning statement that he makes, and I shall quote directly, is this: "One thing that is very noticeable is the loss of the human or personal touch. There is an official air about everything, and every officer is standing on his position and authority. . . . I am much afraid the hospitals are going to consider administrative efficiency and keeping within the rules as being of far greater importance than personal attention to the patient."

This fear is well-founded. That is exactly the situation that prevailed in our own Veterans' hospitals for twenty-five years—administrative efficiency and keeping within the rules were of far greater importance than personal attention to patients. This was not the fault of the doctors; it was the inevitable result of a government bureaucracy.

Again, you might think that this British gentleman is prejudiced against the scheme and consequently can see no good in it. So I shall quote once more from his letter: "Basically, the principle of a comprehensive health service for the nation is as sound as ever, but the practical application of the principle leaves much to be desired." There are the words of a disillusioned man who had expected a better result.

I think these words pretty well express my own convictions upon the question of national health insurance. The theory is most attractive, and I wish ardently that it could be made to work. But I know the elements that are essential to medical care of high quality. I have had to deal with these elements in the medical care of millions of Americans, not daring to lose sight of them for one instant in fashioning the pattern of a medical service. Many of them are intangibles, the existence of which is not suspected by the layman. But they are there, and they are real; and to rush blindly into a new pattern of medical practice, disregarding all psychological considerations as well as administrative obstacles and red lights on the financial horizon, would be only to create a medical system of third-rate quality which, while it might extend the outward forms of medical attention, would offer precious little in the way of good medical care.

I have spoken of rushing blindly into new methods. If you will have the truth, neither the proponents nor the opponents of compulsory health insurance have, at their disposal, enough facts upon which to base final judgment. The only difference between these two factions that is apparent to me is that the proponents of compulsory health insurance appear to regard facts as of little importance. Most of the facts they have so far offered—such as that five million young Americans were rejected for military service in World War II for physical defects that were correctible with medical care, that hundreds of thousands in this country are dying each year because they cannot afford medical care, that there is an appalling inverse correlation between income level and the death rate, that compulsory health insurance has reduced time lost because of illness in those countries in which it is operating—such "facts" as these have been repeatedly exploded. Yet they continue to be offered with no show of embarrassment.

On the other hand, contentions that compulsory health insurance will mean that the Government will take over all doctors and hospitals, that there are no deficiencies in the present pattern of health care and that the practice of medicine is exclusively the business of the doctor are equally insupportable.

This issue of compulsory health insurance has generated a great amount of heat, but a very small amount of light—and it is light that we need before taking such a radical step. I suppose it would be too much to expect, but it would be a most sensible step if the nation could command the services of a nonpartisan and unprejudiced commission of able citizens to explore this matter thoroughly and report facts, instead of guesses and wishful thinking, to our people —a Commission of the general type of the Royal Commissions which have been so useful to the British Government, and of which the recent Hoover Commission is the nearest counterpart in this country.

Thus far, about all that has been collected are rocks, gathered by each side to throw at the other, and some of the contestants seem not to be very particular about the size, shape, or consistency of these missiles. In fact, many of them have been of the consistency of mud.

I may have been guilty of having thrown some of these, myself. If so, I can offer in extenuation of such conduct only that I am intolerant of willful misrepresentation and allergic to politics. There can be no doubt but that some of this controversy has descended to the level of petty politics—a bid for the votes of certain segments of the electorate—and this I deplore. Good health and high quality medical care are too precious assets to become pawns in a political game.

What we need most right now, instead of rocks to be thrown, are nuggets of 24-carat truth, to be weighed in the scale of wisdom. I hope that these will be forthcoming before we arrive at any decision.

To summarize this issue:

1. The quality of medical care in the United States has improved rapidly in the past twenty-five years. This improvement is reflected in many demonstrable ways. We have subdued, if not wholly vanquished, most of the epidemic diseases which have plagued humanity for many centuries. We have increased the average length of life until the high proportion of the aged in our population has created an economic problem of itself. We have greatly reduced time lost from work because of illness. These advances have not ceased, but each year brings further remarkable improvements.

2. These scientific advances, and major changes in our social economy, have increased the cost of medical care to the point where, if it must be met only at the times it is needed, the burden is too heavy to be borne by a considerable part of our people. On the other hand, voluntary insurance, within the reach of almost every self-supporting person, has demonstrated that adequate protection can be had against all but afflictions of long duration; and medical care for such afflictions has long been provided by government for all the population, regardless of income level.

3. There are still deficiencies both in facilities for medical care and in its distribution. Although 98 percent of our population resides within 30 miles of a hospital, there is need for the extension in many areas of facilities for diagnosis. Education, in all fields of the healing art, is in serious need of financial assistance. More preventive medicine is needed. None of these deficiencies, however, is the result of inadequate health insurance. The collections from compulsory health insurance will not finance improvements

in any of these directions. If the government is to do jobs such as these, it will have to finance them by appropriations from the general revenues.

4. In every country in which compulsory health insurance has operated, it has increased the demand for medical care and decreased its quality. Cursory medical attention has had to suffice for careful medical practice. This is not to say that the deterioration of the quality of medical care is an inevitable concomitant of compulsory health insurance; but it is to say that this result is unavoidable when existing facilities are inadequate to meet increased demand. This is the situation at present in the United States. The only way to prevent this deterioration of quality is to provide the added facilities before the demand is increased.

5. More factual information is necessary—both upon the number and magnitude of the deficiencies, and upon the experience of other efforts to eliminate such deficiencies. This information should be collected and evaluated by able citizens whose only concern is the welfare of our people. The issue should be taken out of politics at once.

It should be evident that, with the inadequate amount of knowledge upon the subject that I have at this moment, I am opposed to compulsory health insurance—but perhaps I should have made this clear earlier. However, I hold no convictions that cannot be changed by competent evidence. Thus far, the half-truths and the palpable misstatements that have been advanced to support this radical innovation have failed to convince me. My position is that I recognize the existence of deficiencies to be corrected, but I know of none that cannot be corrected without a radical change in the pattern of medical care—a pattern which has accomplished so much and which continues to raise quality.